what others are saying about
sobrietease

Martha's greatest gift in helping others understand recovery experiences is her use of the written word. Not many are successful weaving their thoughts in a manner so as not to make it about themselves. Martha does this with uncanny wit and brutal honesty. Her clarity into what it means to be part of the largest group of addicts in our nation, while simultaneously being a 40-something recovering alcoholic woman and mother, is refreshing.

Martha is generous in her spirit, raw in her struggle and excited to share her life "behind the velvet rope of Alcoholism" with anyone willing to take a peek. Her foresight to create an honest blog for all addicts and those trying to understand them is a true blessing that reflects just who Martha has become. She is quick to impart to the reader that it is not about her, but rather about living life to the fullest while free from the bondage of addiction. – *Kristin Britt*

All of us go through good times and bad; deal with the flotsam and jetsam of life, small and big. What matters is not whether we have insecurities or weaknesses; whether we make mistakes or just think we've erred. What matters is how we recover from the inevitable "downs" of life, no matter how serious or how devastating those downs can be. Martha Carucci is facing her demons, and helping anyone who reads her blogs to face theirs "out loud." She is showing with grace and humor how to reclaim our lives, how to prevail. Martha prevails. – *Joan Dempsey*

I can personally attest that her blogging has helped hundreds of people in their walk of sobriety, including myself. I love how Martha teaches us to roll with the punches and not take everything so seriously. At the same time, she keeps it real and honest. We always feel better after reading an entry in Sobrietease and we look forward to more.

– *Christy Witschie*

They say you cannot help someone who doesn't want to help themself. Even harder, someone who needed to help themself, but spent their days helping everyone else instead. And did so while battling a demon on a daily basis. Thank you, Martha, for seeing how important you are to us all, and for taking on each day with grace and humor and honesty. You make me laugh, cry, and so grateful that you know you are worth it now.

– *Jenn Hare*

To what depths of despair does one have to fall before realizing that the way up and out depends on your personal strengths and beliefs? Such is what our dear friend Martha has been going through these past few years. Her words will touch and inspire others who yearn for and need some kind of support and guidance on their quests. Martha's writings are forthright and filled with much humor as she has learned that not every circumstance you live through is dire, and the touches of her humanity shine through these pages.

– *Barbara K. Greenfeld*

Martha Carucci has begun a dialog in our community that far surpasses just dealing with addiction. She has opened a can of worms that needed to be opened and has succeeded in bringing so many people together through honest conversation and life sharing. She has helped me, personally, feel that I am not alone with my own issues and obstacles. Her words not only empower and enlighten me, they bring me so much laughter and joy! Thank you, Martha!

– *Tracy Dunn*

Martha Carucci's recovery never fails to amaze me and her blog posts never fail to inspire me. Whether you are in recovery, need to be in recovery or have no problems with addiction, her writing will draw you in. You won't be able to put down her writing pieces once you pick them up!

– Beth Hamilton

Martha Carucci is one of the strongest, most courageous people I know. Not very many struggling with addiction can make the decision to leave it all behind without rehab, but Martha quit cold turkey and threw herself into the program for the good of herself, her children and her marriage. She has been able to channel her energy into her blog, which provides an insight into recovery with humility, honesty, and, of course, Martha's fantastic sense of humor.

Her perspective on life in recovery in the suburbs as a stay-at-home are relatable whether you are on your own path to recovery or just someone in a similar place in life without the alcohol struggles. Her blog resonates in a wonderfully humorous and insightful way. Martha is one funny lady, booze or not.

– Kristin Heidkamp

www.sobrietease.wordpress.com

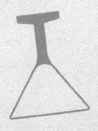

sobrie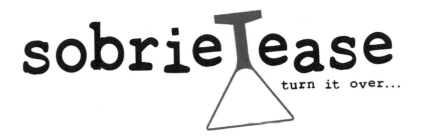ease

turn it over...

martha carucci

God, Grant Me the Serenity to Laugh at Life

Sobrietease
2016

ISBN-13: 978-0-692-68690-4

ISBN-10: 0-692-68690-8

Published by *Sobrietease*
Alexandria, Virginia 22308
www.sobrietease.wordpress.com

Design & Pre-Press by Lucky Valley Press
Jacksonville, Oregon 97530
www.luckyvalleypress.com

Author photo courtesy of Hayden Britt

Sobrietease™ logo designed by J.J. Hogan

Printed in the United States of America on paper that meets
the Sustainable Forestry Initiative® Chain-of-Custody Standards
WWW.SFIPROGRAM.ORG

For my family and for C.H. –
Thanks for being my ray of sunshine every day,
even in the darkest times.

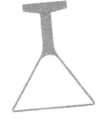

CONTENTS

INTRODUCTION

In 2013, I started a blog called *Sobrietease*. People had been telling me for quite some time that I should start a blog. Why blog? I'm just your average 46-year-old suburban mom. But I have stories to share and lessons to pass on. Many of them are not so average. My problems are no more or less significant than anyone else's—we all have our crosses to bear. I think it is how I have chosen to deal with mine that is worth sharing. Most helpful of all, laughter helps me through the difficult and dark times. I have been given an incredible opportunity—a second chance to live out the rest of my life in much happier and much better ways. My hope is that you will find something somewhere in this book that will strike a chord with you and help you in some way to find yourself in a happier, better place too.

As they say, laughter is the best medicine. It is my new addiction. It may seem heartless to laugh at or mock some of life's most serious trials and tribulations. What's the alternative? I've tried pulling the covers over my head and hiding in my bed several times. I always have to come out for one reason or another. I've tried sweeping everything under the carpet. Works great for a while, until the pile of crap that has been swept under the carpet gets too large and explodes. I've tried to blame others or the circumstances or the way that the planets were aligned at that particular time. I've tried to alter my perception of reality. That worked the best. For a long, long time. And then I woke up and realized that it was, in fact, the worst.

Drinking was a blast. It was a way of everyday life. To me, it was right up there with eating and breathing. Every function, event, celebration, win, loss, mourning, chore, meeting, discussion, creative endeavor, relaxation, motivation...you name it, was not only conducive to drinking, it was centered around it. I was pretty much a happy drunk. Life of the party (or at least I thought I was). With the first sip, my inhibitions and insecurities started to wash away. If one sip allowed that deep exhale of self-doubt and self-loathing to begin to seep out, more sips could only widen the opening and facilitate the escape. That warm, fuzzy feeling came quickly. Not far behind was the ability to throw care to the wind—the "fuck it" period as I liked to call it. All things that should have been done, obligatory crap and responsibilities, took a backseat. I could rationalize anything. You only live once. I'm having fun now, so who cares about anything else. Things looked so much better and brighter. I loved everyone more, especially myself, after the first 750mls worked their magic. It could only go downhill from there. And it did.

I'm reminded of that predictable line at the end of every "Scooby-Doo" episode: I would have gotten away with it too if it wasn't for those meddling kids. There was always a meddling something, most often a nasty hangover involving an unprescribed and unwanted dose of reality. I also thought I was excellent at pretending I wasn't hungover and would act extra chipper on those mornings. Friends who knew me well, however, knew the signs of how bad my hangover was. A single Diet-Coke was usually your average, run-of-the mill hangover. A regular Coke was bad news. Walking around with a plastic cup with a top on it, in case I had to puke was, well, pathetic. It was comical for a while. Even funnier to make it to later in the day when I could dive headfirst into the hair of the dog. And the hamster wheel kept turning.

"No harm, no foul" was the motto I went by. Until things did become more "meddlesome." Appointments were missed either because they were forgotten, not written down, or written down completely illegibly, or because I was simply too hungover to go. Working out wasn't an option when the idea of any sort of physical exertion was equated to doubling over vomiting. I had an unusually frequent occurrence of "headaches," "bad cramps," "stomach bugs," "hangnails"—you name it, that prevented me from doing even basic things.

Conversations were forgotten. Promises made were broken. I was reminded often that I had already told someone something or had done something that I'd already done. All could be excused somehow. The straw that broke the camel's back, however, was when my 10-year-old daughter said to me, "Don't you remember? We talked about that last night?" I don't ever remember feeling more ashamed. That was when I knew things had to change.

And they did.

Martha Carucci
Alexandria, VA
Spring, 2016

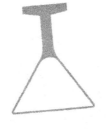

FOREWORD

I don't have a string of letters and titles after my name. There's no MD, PhD, JD, LCSW. So what makes me the least bit qualified to talk about alcoholism and recovery? Because I can add RA to my name, Recovering Alcoholic, and I'm proud to have that title. I also have the distinct honor of being a mother, wife, sister, daughter, friend, sponsee and sponsor. I have over 1,000 days of sobriety under my belt and the number keeps growing. I have lived through and survived the lowest lows of alcoholism and came close to losing everything I had, but now I am winning the battles in the daily Alcoholism War.

I drank to numb. I drank to escape. I drank to celebrate, mourn, relax and to feel better. Name an occasion and I drank to it. It was a way of everyday life. I knew no other way. But the stakes are really quite high in the game of "Let's Take a Drink"- my marriage, family, friendships, health and, ultimately, my life are on the line. My ability to alter my perception of reality and find liquid courage to play the social game worked great... or so I thought, for many, many years. My life was falling apart around me, but I continued to drink. But there was *no way* I was an alcoholic. Not me—an Ivy League-educated, upper-middle class, former lobbyist and suburban mother of three.

Although it is not always easy, I share my struggles and my story openly, hoping that doing so will help others. I got a call today from a friend of a friend who was in a panic. One of her best friends—a wife and mother of two teenagers—had recently been released from rehab and immediately went out, bought wine, and started drinking again. She was irate with everyone for telling her that if she didn't stop drinking, she was going to lose everything. Her husband told her she could no longer live in their home. Hearing this, she stormed out in a fit of rage, saying she would live on the streets. Here was another suburban mother in the throes of the same wretched, powerful disease I have, and it was ruining her life. When they tracked her down, I went to talk to her, calmed her down, and got her to agree to go to a meeting with me and to allow me to be her temporary sponsor.

A few months ago, I got a text from another friend saying she was at her wits' end with her husband and could no longer tolerate his drinking. She asked if I would be willing to talk to him. He was open to her suggestion, as he too faced losing his family and more. He agreed to go to meetings and do an outpatient rehab program. He just got his two-month chip from AA.

On the day I attended my first Alcoholics Anonymous ("AA") meeting, I sat in the car on the phone with my friend who, ironically, lost her husband to alcoholism. I told her I was too scared to go inside. She told me I needed to suck it up and walk in there. She said that there would be people there just like me who wouldn't judge me, and that my life could be so much better than it was. She was right. Why did I listen to her? Because she saw first-hand the effects of alcoholism on others. Why did those two people listen to me? Because I am intimately aware of the effects of alcoholism on the other side.

This book will offer insight to both those who struggle with alcoholism or addiction of any kind and those who care about them, love them and want to help them. By sharing my journey into recovery and through sobriety openly, honestly and humorously, others can seize the opportunity to benefit from my experiences. Alcoholics and addicts can see that it is possible to dig themselves out of that big, dark hole. Family members, friends and loved ones can learn where to find the shovel and other necessary tools and how to support the digging in the most efficient, understanding and beneficial way.

– *Martha*

COMING OUT PARTY

Almost everyone knows someone who is affected in some way by addiction. You may see a bum on the street with a brown paper bag, and have a pretty good idea that he is an alcoholic. But how about the mom sitting at the PTA meeting next to you or watching her child's soccer game in the stands with you? She may be just as miserable, if not more so. We all have our struggles and crosses to bear—whether it's depression, anxiety, addiction of any kind—alcohol, food, drugs, gambling, an abusive relationship, an unhappy marriage—but it's never too late to turn things around. As one of my favorite writers, Brené Brown, says: "Loving ourselves through the process of owning our story is the bravest thing we'll ever do. If we own the story then we can write the ending." Working on owning my story is one of the best things I have ever done for myself.

This book is intended to be a humorous but heartfelt journey about a suburban mom through recovery and sobriety into a better life. Read it and weep, and hopefully laugh.

"If it's sanity you're after,
there's no recipe like laughter."
– Henry Rutherford Eliot

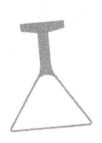

NOW I (AM STARTING TO) UNDERSTAND

One year. 365 days. 8,670 hours. 525,600 minutes. Without a single drop of alcohol. Not one drink. Not even a dose of Nyquil. No mouthwash with alcohol in it. If you had told me on the first day I stopped drinking, Memorial Day of 2012, that I could make it a year, I would have told you that you were insane. As I looked down at my hands shaking, I didn't think I could make it an hour. Yet here I am, one full year later, sober, stronger, healthier, and happier. Some days were easy. Some were hard. Some were downright miserable. And for some I just had to stay in bed. But I did it. I went from shaking to calm. From hungover to energetic. Bloated and heavy, to fit and 15 pounds lighter. From lost to finding myself. Alcoholic to recovering. But still an alcoholic. That will never go away. But I will be a recovering alcoholic with one year of sobriety under my belt, and a shiny coin to carry proudly. Now I understand the will to change and the meaning of endurance.

One year ago today, I woke up in *NYC* (sounds eerily like a Ricky Martin song...) after a late night with some friends on a weekend. I was a strange shade of green, head throbbing, stomach roaring, brain trying desperately to grasp some idea of where I was, what I had done the night before and what was going on. As I started to stir (and probably moan), things began coming back to me in bits and pieces, and I felt my friend take hold of my hand. That simple act meant more to me than any words ever could—that I wasn't alone and that somehow everything would be okay. "The smallest act of kindness is worth more than the grandest intention," Oscar Wilde eloquently penned. One thing I knew for sure was that despite how humiliated, embarrassed, ashamed and badly I felt, there was an enormous weight that had been lifted from my shoulders. My life was going to completely change that morning. It had to. Now I understand why they say "change I must or die I will."

Admitting I had a problem was a huge step for me, and the first move for most people toward any sort of recovery. I knew it deep down and had denied it for so long, rationalizing everything as much as I possibly could to convince myself that I didn't have a drinking problem. It still amazes me how hard it was for me to admit, and amazes me even more that I could ever actually say the words out loud. Some people have admitted their addictions to therapists, doctors, priests, parents, siblings or close friends. I, of course, had to admit it that night in New York to my friend who had recently lost her husband to alcoholism. Great choice, huh? Because why wouldn't someone who endured a horrific battle for two decades with her spouse, but eventually lost, not want to deal with it again with a friend? It would have been completely understandable for her to bail and say, "I just can't do this again," and point me in the right direction to get some help. But she didn't. She told me she would help me through this and has been there every step of the way. She hasn't missed a single day in an entire year of checking in with the same text every morning, "Good morning sunshine, how are you?" Now I understand the true meaning of the word friendship.

As I have said before, everyone has his or her own trials and tribulations and crosses to bear. Sometimes we are strong for our friends. Sometimes we need them to be strong for us. I honestly couldn't have made it to this point in my sobriety without the help of my friends, without their strength, devotion and commitment, and without their confidence in my strength. So to my friends who didn't give up on me, were my wingmen, called me at 5pm on Fridays and went for a walk with me, stocked their fridges with flavored seltzers, literally pulled me out of my bed, made my workout group come chase me down when I tried to hide, convinced me that I was still fun to be around without alcohol, told me they were proud of me, offered to help with my kids so I could get to a meeting, helped get me to focus on other activities that didn't involve drinking, helped me see that life can be so much better and brighter and, despite their fights with their own demons, showed me that they cared and held my hand...thank you from the bottom of my heart. There is a saying I love: "A friend is one that knows you as you are, understands where you have been, accepts what you have become, and still, gently allows you to grow." Now I understand unconditional love.

One year down, hopefully many more to go. But, as they say, one day at a time. Today it's time to stop, breathe and take a minute to pat myself on the back. Now I am starting to understand that it's a choice.

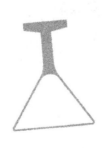

HOW TO...

There's a movie called *How to Lose a Guy in Ten Days*. There are countless magazine articles on "How to Lose 20 Pounds in Two Weeks." *Cosmo* will tell you all sorts of ways of "How to Drive Him Wild," or something like that. I haven't seen much out there about "How to Be Friends with an Alcoholic." Especially one with whom you used to drink incessantly. What happens when booze is no longer part of the equation?

They say in recovery that a changing of the guard is very common with friendships during the transition to sobriety. Yes, it is sad to watch relationships, many of them long-established and seemingly solid, dwindle away, almost like those last ice cubes that sit in the bottom of the glass, melting and mixing in with the final remnants of liquor. There remains only a small puddle of uncertainty and a very diluted relationship. Neither side is quite certain where they stand. The ice has succumbed to the heat and the chemical conversion to its liquid state. The scotch, vodka, gin, whatever, has become watered-down, cloudy and less potent. Sometimes in this mix, it's hard to salvage anything at all.

But there is also the happiness and restored faith that the new guard brings with it. Some of these people may have been there all along, some on the sidelines, the "mixers" if you will, and some brand new. In any case, there's a reason why they are there, right then, at that point in your life. They have moved from the sidelines to the forefront to cheer you on and support you. This is not to say that old is bad and new is good. Remember the saying, "Make new friends, but keep the old, one is silver and the other gold." But there's another expression about not being able to have your cake and eat it too. In order to succeed in sobriety, a person must completely change. In fact, stopping drinking is not necessarily the main part of sobriety. I tried once to stop on my own, and lasted almost a year. By on my own, I mean very little effort and stock put in the program, and barely any of the necessary reflection and self-actualization or mandatory change. Didn't work. Without putting in the work and yes, sometimes sweat and tears, to labor through the twelve steps and change the very core of yourself and what made you drink, it is highly unlikely that you will achieve and maintain sobriety.

But here's the rub: you change. You identify your character defects and work hard to change them. You dig deep down in your heart and your soul, fight with your demons, and hopefully win, and emerge a different but better (and sober) person. Your friends, however, mostly remain the same. Their interaction and involvement in your transition may vary, but for the most part, they aren't going through the same metamorphosis. They look at you, a different person now, through their same eyes. You look at them, the same people, now through your own very different eyes. They may have been the same the whole time and you chose to see them differently, ignoring their flaws, OR missing their strengths and assets. Whatever the vantage point, things are different. A very good friend said to me once, "You can't expect to be completely different and have everything else stay the same." The cake.

So it takes understanding, patience and willingness to learn on both sides. Newly sober, it's difficult to know what to expect from your friends and what they expect from you. Many of them are going through this for the first time as well. Do they continue to drink in front of you? Do they continue to invite you to things where there will be drinking? Do you go even if it's hard for you? Do you decline and stay home, feeling worse for missing out? Or feeling better knowing that you made the right choice for you at the time and did what you had to for your new lifestyle? And that's what it is, a LIFEstyle. Not a phase. Not a trial period. Not the latest 21-day cleanse. A lifestyle.

Here's my advice for both sides (for what it's worth), be honest. Tell each other what you feel comfortable with, and what you don't. Explain to your friends what you need to do to stay sober. If they are interested, tell them how you are working your recovery. Tell them when you just can't do something, and tell them what you can and would like to do. Tell them what's hard. Tell them what works. On the other side, be patient. Ask questions. If the friendship is important to you and worth keeping, remember that this is probably the most difficult thing this person has done in their entire life. Is it hard to be with your old buddy who used to slug down bottles of wine with you on a Tuesday night? I'm sure it is. But, hopefully, the real person inside, without the booze, is a better person to be around, and an even better friend. For some people, it's just too difficult, or too painful, for whatever reason, to continue, and that's okay. Ideally, at the heart of any true friendship is the desire for the other person to be happy and at peace. And if the only way for this to happen is to let them go, then remember this: "God, grant me the serenity to accept the things I cannot change, the courage to change the things I can, and the wisdom to know the difference."

MISS OR MISS OUT?

I miss drinking. I miss everything about it. Well, almost everything. I don't miss the hangovers. Or forgetting stuff. And I don't miss missing out.

I miss the anticipation of that drink, whether it be a nice cold glass of white wine on a hot summer day, or a warm, silky glass of red on a snowy night in winter. Or an ice cold beer on the beach or the golf course. Or a gin and tonic at the end of 18 holes. Don't forget the vibrant pink hue and delightful shape of a Cosmo on a night out with the girls.

I miss going to a friend's house and chatting over a few glasses of wine. I miss going out to dinner and enjoying a bottle of wine that my husband orders.

I miss eating crabs and reaching for a cold beer with my Old Bay-covered fingers.

I miss chasing down spicy Thai food with a lovely, chilled Viognier or Gruner Veltliner.

I really miss the sound of a champagne cork popping and the fizz of the bubbles rising up inside a beautiful crystal flute.

Decaf after dinner is not quite the same as Sambuca and its three floating coffee beans. Or a velvety glass of vintage port. Nowhere close to the taste of Sauternes.

I miss coming up from the beach, putting on music and mixing up some yummy concoctions. The sound of the ice clinking in the glass or being crushed in the blender. Shots of tequila that are like rapidly-fired burning bullets down the hatch. The warmth that quickly spreads throughout the body.

Patterns of behavior. Non-alcoholics may not understand at all, the myriad activities that are associated with drinking. I think about watching a chick flick while my husband is away—I think wine. I want to take a bath to soak aching muscles—I think wine. I think about a wedding—drinking. A funeral—drinking. Theater—pre-theater drinks, intermission drinks, post-theater drinks. Concerts—of course drinking. Skiing—après ski. Bowling—pitchers of beer. Football—tailgates. My kids' lacrosse games—tailgates. Ice skating—hot toddies. Sailing—beers in cozies. Halloween trick-or-treat—road sodas. Christmas—champagne and egg nog. Easter—Bloody Marys. New Years—more champagne. Hanukkah—Manashevitz. Mardi Gras—Hurricanes. The Derby—Mint Juleps. Cinco de Mayo—Margaritas.

Pretty much, if you tried word association with me, I would come up with something alcohol-related for every word. But I don't miss missing out on all the things I did when I was drinking.

I missed out on tucking my kids in and telling them bedtime stories many nights because I passed out early after drinking all day.

I missed out on some great relationships and friendships that crumbled because of my drinking.

I missed out on years I could have been enjoying my marriage.

I missed out on learning many important life lessons because I wasn't listening or couldn't remember them.

I missed out on countless days of just living life because I was too hungover to get out of bed.

I missed out on memories because I blacked out.

I missed out on feeling strong and healthy because alcohol was poisoning my body.

I missed out on knowing that I am worthy of so much more than I believed.

I missed out on pride and self-respect because of things I did when I was drunk.

I missed out on sleeping peacefully through the night.

I missed out on serenity.

But I'm done missing out on life. I am now able to wake up with a clear head, not having to struggle to remember the night before, and realize that every day is truly a gift. I'm missing the drinking less and less with each day of sobriety. No more "miss-takes".

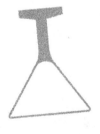

DR. JEKYLL AND MRS. HYDE

Sometimes I'm amazed at how dense I can be. Getting sober has been a great exercise in humility and has opened my eyes to just how much of an idiot I was when I was drinking. But the good news is that for some things, I can say that I wasn't the real idiot, but rather the alcoholism was. I can't use it as a cop-out or to totally absolve myself from the guilt by any means, but it does provide a small cushion. Disease or not, my drinking affected other people.

I brought this topic up in a meeting the other day and it sparked a really interesting discussion. Many women there had examples and stories off the tops of their heads, but others had to do a little memory surfing and really think about how their drinking had affected those around them. Some of them said they remembered things they hadn't thought of in years.

While we were living in our blurred state of being either buzzed or hammered most of the time, we thought that 1) we were absolutely brilliant, hilarious and gorgeous, 2) we were the life of the party, and 3) everyone else around us was probably smashed too, so they wouldn't remember anything stupid we did. But the best delusion was this one: we thought that no one could tell we were drunk. Seriously, think about that. We were slurring, tripping, yelling, carrying-on, singing, pontificating, solving the world's problems with our infinite wisdom, and possibly even falling down or throwing up on someone. But, no, absolutely no one would have known we had been drinking.

I am starting to see how beyond ridiculous it is for me to be surprised or even disappointed when I admit to someone who knows me that I am an alcoholic and their reaction doesn't include the slightest bit of shock. There hasn't really been anyone who has questioned it or said: "You? An alcoholic? No way." The fact that I would even consider that as an option is quite comical. As if their response would be something like this: "I always thought it was completely normal for you to drink several bottles of wine on a random Tuesday night. I mean, who doesn't celebrate Arbor Day like that?" Or, "What kind of ass puts a wall right there where someone can walk smack into it? Clearly a bad floor plan." Perhaps I was expecting something like: "You can't be an alcoholic. I enjoyed telling you the same things over and over and over again and you not remembering them. It was obviously my fault for not telling you in a memorable way."

Instead, it's like a sigh of relief from the other side. Phew. You finally came to your senses. Thank goodness you are getting help. You were a nightmare to deal with when you were drinking. But why does it still surprise me when someone tells me that they knew I had a problem when I thought I did such a great job of hiding it or "acting normal?" I recently talked to a very close friend who told me that upon reading my blog entries, she felt guilty. She felt that she should have done or said something when I was drinking so heavily. She said she was very concerned but didn't know what to do. I told her that even if she had said something to me then, it wouldn't have mattered. I wasn't going to change until I admitted to myself that I had a problem and was ready to face it. That works the other way around too. When one of my friends told me she knew I had a problem, I asked her why she never said anything to me. The answer she gave me was the same. Because it wouldn't have mattered until I was the one who admitted it and was ready to do something about it.

I watched someone this past weekend who, after he got a few drinks in him, completely changed. It was like a totally new person surfaced with the alcohol. I didn't like the new person. There was just a slight edge, cocky, arrogant and a little obnoxious. When I said to my friend that I found this completely unattractive, she pointed out to me that perhaps it was a little like looking in a mirror. How attractive could I have been when I drank and morphed into an entirely different person? Yes, I thought that person was fun, gorgeous, brilliant, etc. But maybe others thought I turned into Mrs. Hyde, and chances are pretty good that they found me completely unattractive as well.

So I started looking back. I looked back at the ridiculous, idiotic and embarrassing things I did when I drank too much. Those actions didn't only have consequences for me, even if it was just waking up with a miserable hangover. They affected other people as well. Other people whose enjoyable night out turned not so enjoyable when they had to hold me up, help me walk, and make sure I got home, the entire time having to endure my senseless babble. They affected other people who were let down the next morning or day when I had to cancel my plans with them because I felt like dirt and spent the day in my bed trying not to puke. And they affected friends, who years later told me that they felt guilty. Guilty that they didn't do anything to help when they knew how much I was drinking. Why should my stupidity and incessant drinking binges be allowed to make someone else feel guilty? Would I have made all those bad choices sober? I think not. But like I said, I can't make the disease the scapegoat. I have to own my actions, process them, make amends where possible and forgive myself.

These friends may not understand that even if they had said or done something, I wouldn't have gotten sober until I was ready to. But they need to understand this: when I was ready to, I did. And knowing that they were there for me then, and are here for me now, means more than I can say (or write).

SOBRIETY ANGEL VS. DRINK DEVIL

It's great to post all these pieces about my come-to-Jesus with myself about my alcoholism, how much better life is sober, how proud I am of myself, etc., but how about when things really just suck and I want a drink? Like now. There are days like this. Luckily they are fewer and farther apart. But they are downright awful.

Holidays are hard for so many people in many different ways. Yes, I realize how incredibly blessed and lucky I am. I don't mean that lightly. I am truly a fortunate person, even more fortunate now that I can see that. My gratitude list is quite long. But still, Thanksgiving for me is very difficult. Ironically, it is my 18-month anniversary to the date. A year and a half of sobriety is nothing to sneeze at, but its significance shrinks substantially when I'm craving a drink. That and many other arguments against picking up seem to have their magic powers zapped from them. That's when the demon of the disease flexes its muscles and tries to take over. I always picture that scene in "Animal House" when Pinto has the little angel on one shoulder and little devil on the other pulling him in different directions. My little angel sits on my shoulder and tells me I would be throwing away 18 months of sobriety, that I would feel terrible the next morning, that I would go back to numbing my way through life, etc. The little drink devil says who gives a flying fuck. It would taste so good. It would take the edge off. It would give me that deep sigh and release. I literally start salivating at the thought of a giant glass of red wine. It's an internal struggle that is completely exhausting.

Thanksgiving was when I stopped drinking the first time, a few years ago. I drank all day and into the evening. I proceeded to have an emotional meltdown in front of my friends and mother, saying some things that I regret to this day. Another Thanksgiving, I don't even remember leaving a friend's house to go home after drinking non-stop. So I should face this holiday tomorrow being thankful for my sobriety and all the wonderful things that come with it. Then how can I sit here and STILL wish I could have a drink? Every practical, rational and sensible reason why I can't indulge in the wines that will be passed around the table with the Thanksgiving turkey are floating in front of my face. Do I swat them away with a rebellious, non-sensible mental fly-swatter? Or do I welcome them and let them permeate my thick-headed skull?

Alcoholism has been described as being "an obsession of the mind" in addition to a "physical addiction." So which is harder to fight? I believe that the physical addiction is overcome earlier in the recovery period. The shakes, the withdrawals, the exhaustion, eventually they go away. The obsession of the mind is another story. Clearly it's still there if I'm talking about wanting a drink 18 months later. However, take one sip of alcohol and it triggers that physical addiction again immediately.

Anything you read about alcoholism will tell you about rationalizing your ability to drink. Maybe I can just drink wine and not hard liquor. Maybe I can just drink beer instead of wine. Maybe I can just drink on the weekends. Maybe I can just drink after 5pm. All of these "abilities," of course, are signs that you are not an alcoholic. Good luck with those. Amazingly enough, that rationalization exists well into your sobriety. Even now I sometimes think that if I have gone this long without drinking, it may now be possible for me to just have one glass of wine. Maybe that first drink won't lead to a zillion others. Maybe, just maybe, I've been "cured" of my alcoholism. Again, dream on.

For those of you who were hoping to read something that would help you get through a day like this, a day when it's just plain hard to not stay in bed with the covers pulled over your head, I wish I had the magic answer. Believe me, I do. The fact that I am writing this at least means that I pulled the covers back off and got out of bed. The fact that I haven't picked up a drink today means that working hard for my sobriety has taught me to reach out to do whatever is necessary—read something helpful, listen to some meditation tapes or just try really, really hard to breathe. To take a deep breath, pray and remember that we do this one day at a time.

YOU! VERSION 2.0: NEW AND IMPROVED! FREE UPGRADE AVAILABLE—ACT NOW!

A good friend of mine calls me "Martha 2.0". The new and improved version. She's seen the old and helped me through the transition, very rough at times, to the new. There will be a version 3.0, 4.0... (eat your heart out Apple). The goal is to keep evaluating, learning, and improving. Find the bugs and problems and fix them. It's a lifelong process. You can upgrade too. It's not exactly free (here comes the fine print): you have to be willing to work for it.

I wish I could explain how clearly I see things now that I'm not drinking. When I drank, it was like I was looking through a pair of glasses with lenses that were covered with water. I could still make things out and see them, but they were usually completely distorted, blurry or just messed up. Occasionally, I would manage to wipe them clean and dry them off, but they would just go back to wet and blurry again. They say the definition of insanity is doing the same thing over and over again, expecting different results. When an alcoholic thinks that they can pick up a drink, and that "this time will be different," they are demonstrating behavior that is, in fact, insane. Every rational, logical and sensible reason why you can't drink is right there in front of you, but so is the insanity of the disease, trying to drop your glasses in the toilet to get wet again.

I had what I considered a sizable breakthrough this week. All it takes is for one person to say something that strikes a chord or zaps a part of your brain to turn a light bulb on. I wish I remembered exactly what they said, but the main point was that they realized that they had to stop blaming someone or something for their drinking. The person, thing or issue didn't CAUSE the drinking. They were just really good EXCUSES to drink, or to continue drinking. I don't believe anyone can maintain sobriety by just stopping drinking. You have to completely change who you are and address the excuses that lead you drink in the first place, especially your own character defects. Work out the bugs. Most importantly, as another wise friend told me, you can't move on until you are willing to lay down the sword when it's time. Letting go of resentments can free up all kinds of memory.

Think about the vicious cycle. As an alcoholic, the problems you experience lead you to pick up a drink. The drinking then, in turn, causes more problems. Things suck more, so you think that drinking will help. It goes on, usually, until you hit rock bottom. Not until you identify and accept the behavior as insanity can you begin to work on improvement. How great would it be if there was some Apple app that "cured" you of alcoholism? One that took away the compulsion to drink. An app that let you skip the horrible withdrawal and expedite recovery. An incredible app that fixed everything you screwed up when you drank. Unfortunately, there isn't. The tools at your disposal are the experience and understanding of those who have been through this before you. Those who have worked hard to achieve and maintain sobriety. If you are willing to do the work and use these tools, you too can get your upgrade. Act now. It's vital to be plugged in during the process. Hooking up to your HP (Higher Power) usually works best. And there's also a holiday two-for-one special going on now—help someone else up and you will help yourself at the same time.

TAKE A DRINK, I USED TO THINK

It would solve it all, I used to think
To simply pour and pick up a drink

A tall glass, a short glass, I really didn't care
As long as enough booze was floating in there

The first little taste that touched on my lips
Was followed by many, many more sips

Vodka and soda, tonic and gin
As much and as many as I could fit in

What's the big deal, I was totally fine
I'd move from the hard stuff right over to wine

Before very long, one glass became four
Another bottle opened to continue the pour

Things seemed so much brighter and lighter and free
I could step far away and not have to be me

An escape, what a treat, what a break from it all
Higher and higher I would build up the fall

My bed was my haven, my solace from life
No pressure, no let downs, no more of the strife

No trying to please, no worry, no cares
No fighting, no fearing or threatening stares

The haven would spin, more often than not
Wishing, again, I hadn't had that last shot

I'd wake up and wonder what I did, where I was
I had no idea since my brain was just fuzz

My mouth really dry, head pounding and dull
As if someone threw a big brick at my skull

The day would be long, I knew right away
But all who would see me would think I'm okay

All chipper and smiley, no hangover for me
Is what those who saw me would usually see

But those who knew better were used to my game
Though they still couldn't see through to the guilt
    and the shame

How long can I go living life in this way?
Drinking and wasting every single damn day

You can numb and ignore it for only so long
Then the true test will come to see if you're strong

Strong enough to be humble, to admit that you know
That the path that you're on isn't the right way to go

You've finally come to that fork in the road
Struggling and trying to hold on to your load

You throw down your pride at last to the ground
Finally listening to the absence of sound

If you can only be silent, and open your ears
You can now finally start to face all your fears

It's really quite simple, it's hard to believe
That life is no more than a daily reprieve

Admit you are powerless, you've lost your control
Of every last bit that remained of your soul

If you're willing to do this and choose the right path
Someday you might find you'll be able to laugh

And smile again, in a genuine grin,
Not like in the stupor you used to be in

Many of those who have struggled before
Are right there to help you, they're holding the door

And the one thing I leave you, my wisdom to share
If you open your heart, your God will be there.

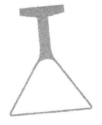

THE POWER OF PRAYER
(AND A PINT OF BEN AND JERRY'S)

Several years ago, I was seated next to a woman at a birthday dinner for a friend. I knew her, but not well. I had heard she was going through a rough separation with her husband but didn't know the details. She had three small children and when I had seen her occasionally around the neighborhood, she looked like she had been through the ringer. During our conversation, she opened up and told me about her situation. It was a terrible story that involved her husband having a drug addiction she was unaware of and spending most of their savings, getting deeper and deeper in debt to his habit. As I listened in disbelief and sympathy, I asked her how in the world she got through it. She told me that she didn't get through it alone. She said that she felt as though someone, or something, picked her up and helped her to be able to carry on with each day to do what she needed to for her children and herself. She told me that she felt God's presence and that she was convinced that it was He who provided her with the strength she needed at her worst hour. Having had several cocktails already, I tried to keep myself from outwardly displaying through facial expressions or body language that I thought she was completely nuts. Um, yeah, ok…some strange force picked you up and carried you through your day. And I suppose there were little green men helping you push your shopping cart at the grocery store as well.

After that night, I think I only saw her one other time. I heard that she and her husband reconciled, that he got help and was able to beat his addiction, and they managed to keep their family together. They also spent a great deal of time focusing on their faith and good fortune, which they believed was brought to them by God. I didn't think about this woman for years, until recently. And I can honestly say that now I get it. I completely understand what she meant when she said that something much greater and more powerful than anything she had ever known lifted her up and carried her until she could stand again on her own two feet.

Growing up, the extent of my religious practices involved reluctantly going to church on Christmas and Easter and trying to stay awake. I knew nothing about the Bible, Christianity, or theology. More importantly, I knew nothing about spirituality, or the fact that spirituality and religion are two completely separate things. After getting married in the Catholic church, and especially after our children were born, I started to attend church much more regularly. But still, only when things got rough, or when dealing with the loss of a loved one, did I turn my glance upwards, mostly looking for answers. Then there were the many times, usually while paying homage to the porcelain god after a night of mixing drinks, that I either asked God to help me stop feeling so sick or vowed to Him that I would never drink again. That never lasted very long.

When I took my last drink almost 21 months ago, the realization that I could never, ever pick up a drink again was beyond overwhelming. It seemed downright impossible. Add to that the knowledge that no one could do this for me, or really do anything to help but be there to support me, and that's more than rubbing salt in the wound. There was no magic pill that a doctor could prescribe. There was no therapist who could magically remove the compulsion to drink. There was no trainer, life coach, personal assistant, clergy, shaman, or magic wand. There was only me. And, when I was ready to know, understand and trust it, my Higher Power (HP).

I often think that if I only knew when raising my first child what I now know while raising the third, my life would have been so much calmer. But as they say, hindsight is 20/20. While I was immersed in diapers, nursing, bottles, spit-up, and sleepless nights, I couldn't see that if I only took a deep breath and calmed down, I could have enjoyed that precious time alone with a beautiful new life. By the time I got to my third child, I wasn't obsessed about sanitizing a pacifier after it fell to the ground, or as much of a sleep-Nazi about nap time and schedules. He got thrown into his car seat, whatever time of day, to shuttle the other two kids around to their activities. He had to just go with the flow. In fact, I would often just put the baby down for a while in his little playpen and just let him be…without hovering over him to make sure he was still breathing every few minutes!

Similarly, if I had only known during those first few weeks of sobriety what I know now, it would not have been quite as torturous. Don't get me wrong, it still would have been pure hell, but the knowledge I have now certainly would have helped. Admitting having a life that is unmanageable due to an addiction to alcohol is the first huge step. Understanding that you cannot fully recover from that addiction without turning to, and relying on, your HP is the next crucial turn. That's the magic bullet. The power of determination helps. The power of friendship and support helps. The power of inner strength helps. But the power of prayer heals.

When I started to understand that if I was willing to turn my will and my life over to the care of God, the road to recovery would be much smoother. There will still be many bumps and potholes, but that belief and willingness helps to pave a smoother path. I used to sit in church and during the quiet prayer time after communion, I would hold my head in my hands and cry silently. I was miserable. And usually hungover as it was a Sunday morning. I positioned myself physically as far away from anyone, including my family, as I possibly could, even in the same pew. I didn't want to make eye contact with anyone. I chose to sit and drown in my depression. I asked God for help. But it didn't come. Not on my terms anyway…

As I learned more and more during my recovery, and truly trusted in turning things over to my HP, I started to see the magic at work. I noticed that somehow I would hear something from a friend (angel?) on a day when that was exactly what I needed to hear. And I actually was listening for a change. I realized that the people who surrounded me where there for a specific reason. A kind word of support or pat on the back worked wonders for my will to fight on. I saw that the fortuitous encounter with a well-respected pastor with whom I shared my story recently was probably no accident.

I have prayed for strength for my recovery and I am still sober, 626 days later. I have prayed for support and understanding from family and friends and I have that. I have prayed for healing and learning to forgive myself and I am on the right path. I have prayed for guidance with some tough situations and have gotten it. I have prayed for the ability to sit quietly and listen and I'm getting better at that. Sometimes I will need a kick in the head to remember to turn to prayer and my HP when things get really rough, but hopefully I will get that kick too from the people who care about me and whom God has put in my life to help me. As for the pint of Ben and Jerry's, that can help immensely as well.

SERENITY TO LAUGH T-SHIRT IDEAS

In keeping with my tagline "God, Grant Me the Serenity to Laugh at Life"...here are some new *Sobrietease* t-shirt/bumper sticker ideas I've come up with:

Jose Cuervo – I Kicked Your Ass

Ben and Jerry Can Kick the Shit Out of Bartles and James

I Got My Memory Back-ardi

Margarita Was a Ho

Jack Daniels is for Sissies. Real Men Drink Fresca.

Absolut Jackass

I Stoli Your Hangover

Captain Morgan Was a Wuss

I'll Have a Martini, Hold the Gin. And the Vermouth...
Screw It—Just Give Me a Bowl of Olives

Manhattan? Try a Harlem Instead

Bloody Mary? Gee That Sounds Good...NOT

7 & 7 Equals Coke Zero

Water – The New 'It' Drink

It's 8am Somewhere

Kiss Me I'm Sober

I Lost My Mohijo

Sober. The New Drunk (heard this one from a friend)

Why Don't We Not Get Drunk and Screw Tonight?

Do You Want Salt and Lime With That Seltzer Shot?

Fuzzy Navel? TMI

Holy Shit! Is That What You Really Look Like??

I Wasn't a Blackout Drinker... As Far As I Can Remember...

TURN THE BEAT AROUND

I was listening to one of my favorite church songs this morning during Easter mass. It's called "The Bread of Life" and for some reason, every time I used to hear it, I would cry. It wasn't the words of the song that brought out the tears—it's a happy song which basically says that those who believe in Jesus will want for nothing and be raised up to live forever. Clearly, it wasn't the song. It was what was going on in my life at that time that made me cry. Today, I listened and smiled with my kids next to me and I started thinking about music and what a huge role it plays in our lives.

You can hear a song and it can instantly take you back to a particular time, event, or memory. Driving back from Charleston yesterday—a lovely 10-hour car ride with a sick husband, my daughter with her headphones permanently affixed to her head, and my two boys acting out the WWF championships in the back seat, I heard everything from classic rock to 70s and 80s tunes to Country Music. Looking at the lyrics of the songs you listen to through the decades and stages of your life says a great deal about you.

In elementary school, I enjoyed the deep, philosophical lyrics of artists (and I use that term very loosely) like Sheena Easton, Rick Springfield, Adam Ant, Men at Work, Taco, Loverboy, Sammy Hagar, Duran Duran, Human League...I could go on. We didn't know any better to realize that most of these lyrics made no sense or were completely stupid. Who the hell was Jessie and why do we care about his girl? If I had a nickel for every time someone dialed 867-5309, I'd be up there with Bill Gates and Oprah in Forbes. And come on, Eileen, drive your little red Corvette to see your friends Mr. Roboto and Mickey, who is so fine that he blows minds. When you get there, you can do the Stray Cat Strut or the Safety Dance, all while putting on the Ritz. Deep. Very deep.

I got into high school and learned that Whitney wanted to dance with somebody and George Michael wanted your sex. To which Debbie Gibson replied "only in my dreams." Huey was doing it all for his baby while the Beastie Boys fought for their right to party. Poor, abused Luka got lost in emotion with Lisa Lisa and Cult Jam. Bananarama heard a rumor that Madonna was on La Isla Bonita and the lady in red went to the land of confusion with Genesis. And sorry Gloria Estefan, but the rhythm never did get me. At this moment, no sign of Billy Vera and the Beaters. But some of those songs became important to us as prom themes, background noise to first kisses, or party music while we tried to be cool and shotgun beers in dark woods tucked inside a local golf course.

College brought a more worldly and sophisticated array of music. The British invasion gave us New Order, the Smiths, the Cure, Depeche Mode and many others. It was so cool to listen to that ever-cheery Morrissey crooning things like "if a ten-ton truck crashes into us, to die by your side is such a heavenly way to die" and "sweetness I was only joking when I said by right you should be bludgeoned in your bed." If that didn't lead to heavy drinking, I don't know what did. Marky Mark sang about good vibrations while REM complained about losing their religion. DNA featuring Suzanne Vega gave us *Tom's Diner*, which once we got in our heads, we couldn't stop singing all day. How Gerardo's "Rico Suave" didn't walk away with the highest accolades of the music industry is beyond me. I guess Vanilla Ice gave him some stiff competition. Oh, and Milli Vanillli, how devastated were we when we found out that they were lip-synching frauds? Blame it on the rain, I want to be rich. Crushing.

It wasn't until recently that I found myself leaving the country station on the radio a little longer. Some great music and talented artists. But I think I have to say that of all the music I have listened to over the decades, no genre features songs about alcohol more than country. Of course you will find songs about drinking in other genres. George Thorogood had to have his one bourbon, one scotch and one beer. Jimmy Buffett sang about *Margaritaville* and *Boat Drinks*, and reminded us that it's 5 o'clock somewhere. Even my favorite opera, *La Traviata*, has the drinking song where Alfredo and Violetta belt out in beautiful Italian *"libiamo –let's drink, let's drink in joyful chalices…let's enjoy the pleasures, fleeting and fast."* One of Broadway's most brilliant offerings, *Les Miserables*, includes a song called *"Drink With Me."* I would drink nonstop too if I were Jean Valjean.

But as I started listening more carefully to the titles and lyrics of country songs, I saw a very common theme. Here are just a few examples of song titles:

Drink in My Hand - Eric Church
Drinks After Work - Toby Keith
Drink One for Me - Jason Aldean
Drink a Beer - Luke Bryan
The More I Drink - Blake Shelton
Save Water, Drink Beer - Chris Young
Get My Drink On - Toby Keith
I Like Girls That Drink Beer - Toby Keith
Drink on It - Blake Shelton
Haven't Had a Drink All Day - Toby Keith
Drink One More Round - Cory Morrow
Drink Too Much - Mark McKinney
Drink Your Whiskey Down - Reckless Kelly
Drink More Beer - Rodney Carrington
Drink, Drank, Drunk - Cowboy Troy

The World Needs a Drink - Terri Clark
Two Rounds of Jose Cuervo - Tracy Byrd
Two Pina Coladas - Garth Brooks
And...
Why the Hell Do You Think I Drink? - Joe Nichols

And that is just a small sampling. Some of those songs are pretty funny, some are sad, and some just raise red flags that their writers should consider a stop in at the Betty Ford Clinic their next time out on tour. In my continued journey in sobriety, I tend to enjoy listening to the songs that talk about someone's life going down the crapper from drinking. They remind me of the benefits of sobriety. The station gets changed quickly for all the songs romanticizing alcohol. As things get better in my life with each day sober, I don't find myself crying at songs as much. I don't even need Bobby McFerrin to tell me not to worry and to be happy, or have to play Pharrell to dance around "happy." It comes more often and more naturally. Maybe I should work on my own song—something to the tune of one day at a time, life is a hell of a lot better sober. Hmmm...

To paraphrase the words of the iconic Swedish band Abba, thank you for the music and all the joy it brings.

TO MY FAMILY ON MOTHER'S DAY

It's Mother's Day again, that very special day
We all like to celebrate in our own unique way

Some moms like to spend the day on their own
Some time to regroup, some time all alone

Some go for a picnic in the park with their clan
Some wait for their kids to come up with a plan

Their husbands go out and buy them a gift
Hoping their efforts will give mom a lift

A nice dinner out so we don't have to cook,
One day of the year we are let off the hook

Cold coffee and burnt toast delivered in bed
A construction paper crown placed upon my head

Last year was a brewery for Mother's Day lunch
Not the plan this year, that's just my hunch

This year I'll be sober for almost two years
The last thing I'd like is to be surrounded by beers

Flowers are nice, and jewelry is too
But what I actually want, they haven't a clue

It's really quite simple, I think you'll agree
A small list of things you can all do for me

Take out the garbage, pick up your crap
Stop screaming and fighting while I try to just nap

Put your dishes in the sink, or even better yet,
The dishwasher would be a much smarter bet

What's that? How do you know if it's dirty or clean?
I'll tell you it's easy, and I don't mean to be mean

Just open the damn door, and take a good look
Are they shiny and clean or covered in gook?

What other questions keep you from doing your part?
Ask me what you need to, I'm really quite smart

Where is the vacuum? Where is the broom?
It's not that hard, they're in the same room.

You can't put things away, where do they go?
If you try really hard, I think you'll see that you know

You can't reach? It's too high to put that away?
Let me introduce you to your friend Mr. Stepladder today.

But where should I put my lax stick? My ball? My glass?
You know where you can put them? Right up your...

Put your dirty clothes in the hamper, your clean clothes away
And no, that's not dirty, you wore it for 5 seconds today

Picking up doesn't mean shove it under your bed
Or hide it away in your closet instead

You ask for a dog, a cute little puppy,
But you can't even take care of our poor stinking guppy

It swims in its tank, all covered in green
Waiting for someone to make it all clean

I'll get right on that, as soon as I'm free,
2026 looks like that's when I may be

Put away the cereal, the milk and the bread
No, don't leave it out "for the next person" instead

Just once do your homework, without being told
Over and over, it gets really old

I'm tired of tripping over your boots and your shoes
The fact that we have closets is really old news

Oh no, by all means, leave those chips on the floor
I'm sure I saw that look featured in this month's Elle Decor

A bubble bath and a candle and a nice little snack
With little green army guys digging into my back

Or a night on the couch with popcorn and a movie
That gum stuck under the cushion sure feels really groovy

Ok, you know what would be a really good goal?
My friends Ben and Jerry filled up in a bowl

I'll just go to the kitchen and get it myself
But wait, there isn't a clean bowl to be found on the shelf

They're all in the dishwasher covered in food
It hasn't been run, now here goes my mood

I'll just get a spoon and eat the whole thing
I'd rather have ice cream than any more bling

So I open the freezer - the ice cream has all been eaten
For Mother's Day there will now be a nice family beatin'

I can live without clean floors or a nice empty sink
But there is one thing that will push me right over the brink

You ate my damn ice cream, my Mother's Day prize
I was really looking forward to it going right to my thighs

That was the last straw, a low blow, a slap in the face
A trip to the spa, now that may be the right place

Just go play your Minecraft, your Sims and your Wii
Don't worry at all about Mother's Day for me

You're really good kids, and I am a lucky mom it's true
Now go play in the street before I ground you.

WEAK ENOUGH

For some reason, things get a little slippery for me around anniversaries. Many people have told me that they have the same issue. Not sure what it is. I'm coming up on my two-year anniversary on May 28th. God willing, I will have made it 730 days, one day at a time, without a drink. Why, when I can practically taste the sweetness of my accomplishment, would I even entertain the thought of picking up a drink now? Is it easier to sabotage my own success than have to worry about continuing the daily battle?

When I shared today that I was feeling scared, doubtful and uncertain about whether I had the strength necessary to maintain a sober life, someone told me something that really stuck. "It's not about whether you are strong enough. It's about whether you are weak enough. Weak enough to realize that you can't do this yourself, but that God can. Weak enough to turn it over." It gave me a whole new way to look at things. It's okay to be scared. In fact, it's good to be scared and show your humility and respect for the fight for sobriety. I've done cocky too. I got this. No problem. Somewhere in between there's a happy medium—or as my friend calls it, "The right size box."

So back to where I was…scared, doubtful and uncertain. What helps now is going back to basics. One day at a time. If I have to, one hour at a time. Remembering all the things in my life that are so much better now that I am sober. Thinking about the stupid mistakes I made when I was drinking. Remembering how good I feel now, physically and emotionally, and how bad I felt Before Sobriety. I'm gonna call it "B.S." I don't want to go back to B.S.

Often when a new year is approaching, people create "In and Out" lists—what is going out of style and what is coming in for the approaching year.

So here is my in and out list, or B.S. vs. A.S. list:

B.S. (*OUT*)	A.S. (*IN*)
Resentment	*Compassion*
Insecurity	*Humility*
Depression	*Security*
Anger	*Pride*
Low Self-esteem	*Joy*
Doubt	*Happiness*
Weakness	*Understanding*
Fear	*Strength*
	Confidence

Which list do you think looks better? Whether it's two years, two decades or two hours of sobriety, what separates us is only one second. The second before we pick up a drink or not. So in that one single second, pray that you are weak enough. That's my plan.

TURN THE BEAT AROUND, PART II

After my post "Turn the Beat Around," a good friend of mine, who happens to be a huge country music fan, sent me a nice note. She said while she liked it, "to defend her love of country," I had to "give country music some accolades for recognizing addictions too." Sounds totally fair. She gave me just a few examples of songs I should check out. Yes, she was right. In my other piece, I wrote a long list of songs romanticizing drinking. In deference to my friend, here are a few examples of country songs that really capture the evils of addiction:

"That's Why I'm Here"—Kenny Chesney—"The devil takes your hand and says no fear. Have another shot, just one more beer." The devil loves alcohol and the chaos that comes with it. This song goes on to talk about the simple things in life and the risk of losing them all to alcohol.

"Choices"—George Jones—talks about "living and dying with the choices I've made."

It is your choice. And you can either choose to live, or choose to drink and die.

"Some People Change"—Montgomery Gentry—a salute to the "strong and brave" and encouragement to not give up hope because people do change. He also thanks God for the ones who have made it out of the darkness of addiction and urges them to be the "Light".

And there are many more. Those are just a small sampling. I have to admit, that's good, powerful stuff. Thank you to my friend for sharing those with me. In response to the songs above, I agree people do change. I'm a living, breathing example of that. We all live and die with the choices we make. Dr. William Glasser, the psychiatrist who developed the "choice theory" said that "it is almost impossible for anyone, even the most ineffective among us, to continue to choose misery after becoming aware that it is a choice." There is way too much for me to say about choice here, that's for another post on my blog. For now, suffice it to say that I choose to stay sober and I choose happiness. And yes, I choose to agree that country music ain't so bad.

CONSIDER IT PURE JOY

I had never even opened a bible. Perhaps I looked at one or two sitting in nightstand drawers at hotel rooms. That's about it. I participated in my first bible study at the same time I started my battle against alcoholism, a little over two years ago. A friend asked me to join her, thinking it would be a good idea to get me to turn my attention to activities that didn't involve drinking. While I didn't know too much about bible studies, I was pretty sure they didn't involve sitting around doing tequila shots every time someone said the word "Jesus." It was amazing how much the two things were compatible and reinforced each other. In my twelve-step program, I was learning about the need to turn to faith in order to achieve and maintain sobriety. The bible study taught me the need to turn to faith in order to achieve and maintain sanity and grace.

The study focused on the book of James, which has been described by Bible Hub as "a book about practical Christian living that reflects a genuine faith that transforms lives." A good place for a bible newbie to start, and an excellent place for someone seeking transformative faith to start. I'll never forget one of the first lines of the book of James: "Consider it pure joy, my brothers and sisters, whenever you face trials of many kinds, because you know that the testing of your faith produces perseverance." My personal translation was this: "Be glad that you are going through living hell because it will make you stronger." In other words, what doesn't kill you makes you stronger and there is a reason for it. Whatever your struggle, there is a reason behind it and somehow, someway, even though we may have a hard time seeing it or understanding it, God has a plan and will produce some good from it.

With the bible study homework, I did a fair amount of soul-searching. This is going to be great, I thought. I can't wait to figure out just how the hell my decades of alcoholic drinking, blackouts, falling down stairs, etc., would bring about something good. So far, all I could figure out was that it got me to open a bible and to meet some very interesting women. Not to mention the fact that I went to an activity from which I emerged as sober as I was when I arrived.

But I noticed that while I started to read "the word," worked on turning my will and my life over to God (Step Three), and simply became more present in my life by being sober, I began seeing "God-winks" all around me. Squire Rushnell has an excellent book called *When God Winks at You*, all about certain "chance" circumstances that can only be explained by divine intervention (God-winks).

I started writing a blog about my journey through recovery. The more I wrote, the more cathartic it was, and the more it helped in my soul-searching and self-awareness. People started to comment about my blog, pull me aside and tell me that they shared it with their friend/mother/father/cousin/uncle/aunt/brother/sister/butcher...anyone they knew struggling with addiction. The more I heard, the more I realized how much addiction touches almost everyone in some form or shape, and the more I wanted to help.

There were several other God-winks, but one of the biggest came on a Sunday morning when I grabbed my coffee and turned on the television. I flipped it to the well-known evangelist, Joel Osteen, at the exact time he was saying these words: "God can take your mess and turn it into your message. God knows how to use what you've been through. He doesn't waste any experiences. He can use what you've been through to help others in that situation. Nothing is wasted, the good, the bad, the painful." It was as though he was speaking directly to me. It strongly reaffirmed my feeling that I am supposed to take my mess, my bad, my pain and not waste it, but rather use it to help others in a similar situation. That situation doesn't have to be alcoholism. It can be whatever trial or tribulation you suffer in your life. It reinforced the fact that it's never too late to change something bad into something good. To consider it pure joy.

Another major God-wink came in the form of an opportunity a few weeks ago to speak to women in a local jail. It was a small group of women in what they called the "Sober Living Unit," who had committed to try to live a clean and sober life when they left their incarceration. I had no idea what to expect, and even less of an idea what I was going to say. But somehow, the words just came. God gave me the guidance and the words I needed.

I began by telling my story, and then went on to share two pieces from my blog, which were very well-received. At the end, there was no awkward silence as I feared, but rather an extensive, interactive discussion. Each woman shared some of her story, but not all explained what they had done to land themselves in this dreadful place. Several were there for selling drugs. One woman drank so much that she passed out with her small child next to her, only to be awakened by a police officer and arrested for child abandonment/neglect. That prompted me to share the story of a friend of mine who had relapsed twice after brief periods of sobriety, each time with major repercussions. The first time, she picked up a drink simply because it was a nice, sunny, spring day. She finished a bottle of vodka and decided to drive to the ABC store to get more. She realized she was in no shape to be driving, pulled over and passed out in her car. She, too, was awakened by police officers, and lost her license for a year for driving under the influence. The second time, she drank so much after being upset by an argument that she again passed out. This time she woke up to find police and Child Protective Services at her door because someone had called saying that the children were alone with an incapacitated mother. Two relapses. Two major screwups. But her mess turned into my message. God didn't waste it. Does she consider it pure joy? I doubt it. But perhaps just one of those women will remember it when they return to their normal lives and think twice about picking up a drink or selling drugs.

The entire time, I was well aware of how incredibly blessed, and lucky, I am. But for the grace of God, I could be in there with them myself. Have I driven when I shouldn't have? Yes. Have I been incapacitated around my children? I'm so incredibly ashamed to admit yes. All the more reason why I feel strongly about my need to make what they call living amends. I have been given the chance to live my life in a much better and healthier way, so why wouldn't I take that and use it in the best ways I can? I'm in no position to preach or give advice, but I told the women as I was leaving that it was not too late for them to change and turn their lives around. They have to start in there as we do out here, one day at a time.

The book of James also includes what I like to call the "Put Your Money Where Your Mouth Is" message. "Do not merely listen to the word, and so deceive yourselves. Do what it says. Anyone who listens to the word but does not do what it says is like someone who looks at his face in a mirror and, after looking at himself, goes away and immediately forgets what he looks like." Sometimes it's really hard to look in the mirror. Often we don't like what we see. Look. Really look. Listen and act. Read and do. James also says "faith, by itself, if it is not accompanied by action, is dead... Show me your faith without deeds, and I will show you my faith by my deeds." I have faith that I can stay sober. But if that faith is not accompanied by action, by hard work, rewiring and praying, it is dead. For a relatively short bible book, James contains so many other powerful messages. "Everyone should be quick to listen, slow to speak and slow to become angry." Quick to listen and slow to speak. Advice everyone could benefit from. And "the tongue is a small part of the body, but it makes great boasts. Consider what a great forest is set on fire by a small spark." There is so much good stuff in here. Why didn't I pick up this book in the hotel rooms?

Finally, the last chapter of James leaves us with this: "...if one of you should wander from the truth and someone should bring that person back, remember this: Whoever turns a sinner from the error of their way will save them from death and cover over a multitude of sins." I'm not sure I have the power to bring someone back from sin or wandering in the wrong direction. I have to start with myself. However, I have a friend, an older woman, who is a very nervous driver and gets completely frazzled when people behind her are driving too close. She called me over to her car in the parking lot one day after a meeting and said she wanted to show me something. There, taped on her steering wheel, was a piece of paper with a simple message and reminder to herself: "Consider it pure joy."

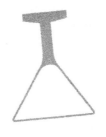

PAY IT FORWARD

When I was a college student in Philadelphia, a good friend and I would occasionally venture downtown to take in a little culture with a concert by the Philadelphia Orchestra. The Academy of Music often made student tickets available just a few minutes before the concert was about to start. On one occasion, Midori, the famous young violinist, was scheduled to perform. We knew that chances were very slim that we would be able to get tickets as the concert would likely be sold out. We decided to give it a shot and at least enjoy a nice dinner in the city and try our luck.

When we got to the box office, just as we thought, the performance was completely sold out. No student tickets, or any other tickets for that matter, were available at all. As we turned to go on our merry way and head back to campus, an elegantly dressed old woman approached us. She was apparently waiting for a friend who never showed. "You look like a nice young couple," she said. "Would you like my tickets?" My friend politely asked her how much she wanted for them, expecting the price to be much higher than we could afford. "Nothing" she replied. "Perhaps one day when you are my age, you will do the same thing for someone else." We gratefully took the tickets, thanked the woman profusely and found our seats. Sixth-row center. They didn't get much better than that. They would have cost a fortune, at least for two college students.

The concert was beautiful and Midori's playing was simply magical. For about two hours, I wasn't a college student in the throes of exams and stress. I was a million miles away, escaping to a peaceful, melodic haven. I couldn't help think throughout the entire concert about the woman who gave us the tickets. Who was she waiting for? Why didn't they show up? Why didn't she stay and enjoy the concert herself? Did she leave the box office feeling lonely and disappointed by being stood up? Or was she happy knowing that her kindness brought some much needed peace and respite to two young students? I closed my eyes, listened to the glorious sounds of the violin and orchestra, and pondered all of those things. Her misfortune turned into our fortune. Another God-wink? Perhaps.

I'm not sure there is a better representation of the expression "pay it forward." Will my friend or I, or both of us, do the same for someone else some day? Yes. Here it is, more than twenty years later, and I remember that night, and the natural high it brought, like it was just yesterday. I hope that when I am her age, I'm not standing alone waiting on someone who never comes. I hope I continue to hear the beautiful music. And I hope that night ended peacefully for her, with a simple explanation for why her friend never came. But if I do find myself in the position to pay it forward, I most certainly will. When we open our eyes, we can see the God-winks all around us. And sometimes, God places the "winks" in our own hands to do with them what we will.

As Plato said, *"Music gives a soul to the universe, wings to the mind, flight to the imagination and life to everything."*

A pretty amazing thing to pay forward.

EXTRA! EXTRA! DRINK ALL ABOUT IT

The news these days is nothing short of devastatingly depressing. The terror group ISIS is beheading innocent people and trying to instill fear and horror throughout the world. The deadly Ebola virus is spreading at an exponential rate. There is a terrible respiratory illness that is sending hundreds of children to emergency rooms nationwide. Nationally recognized and idolized sports figures are being exposed for brutally beating their partners and even their children. Ugh.

So when we are bombarded from every direction with negativity, fear and sadness, what do we do? Everyone has their own way of dealing with difficult times, their own coping mechanisms. Some meditate, many pray, some repress it and continue on, some seek help, some shut down and, if you're an alcoholic, chances are you drink. It's usually the only coping mechanism you know. If you're a recovering alcoholic, you may struggle to refrain from picking up a drink.

I can only speak about my own experiences and feelings as an alcoholic. Thank goodness I am an alcoholic in recovery who hasn't had a drink in over 2 years (845 days to be exact). With each day that I am inundated with bad news however, the brick wall that I have been building, one day at a time, to protect me and keep me away from the bottle, gets chipped away. It's like a chisel is breaking out little holes through the wall that give me glimpses of past coping mechanisms in the form of liquid. There's a tiny voice in the back of my head that tries to tell me that with all these horrible things that surround me, what the hell could be so bad about taking a drink? My brain still fights the many years of training that taught it that when things were tough, I could always pick up a drink and feel better. The insanity of the disease of alcoholism tries to tell me that a drink will wash all my cares away.

The reality, however, is quite harsh. A drink will not destroy ISIS, cure Ebola or deadly respiratory illnesses, stop domestic violence, or bring a missing girl home. A drink will do absolutely nothing to help make things better. Absolutely nothing. Not only will it do nothing to make things better, it will make things worse. Much worse. I've had crappy days when I have wanted to have a drink. I've also had wonderful days, when all seems right with the world, or my little world anyway, when I have also wanted to pick up a drink. Good times, bad times, happy times, sad times, a drink seemed appropriate for all. But it was never "a" drink. It was a drink followed by another drink, and then another, and then another...I like to explain my alcoholism to people as a broken switch in my brain wiring. I believe that "normal" people have a little light that comes on in their brain that tells them they have had enough to drink and need to stop. The little switch is flipped and they make the rational, prudent decision not to drink any more at that time. In my brain, the light, and the switch, are either broken or missing. As I approach too much to drink, instead of telling me to stop, my brain tells me to keep on going. More is better.

What scares the hell out of me now is that if I can crave a drink at times when things are going well, how in the world am I going to resist a drink when something really difficult happens? And not just out in the world, but to me, or in my immediate little world. An integral part of recovery is breaking down your ego and your self-centeredness. When I drank, it was all about me. First and foremost. ME, where my next drink was coming from, when I was getting my next drink, what was going to make ME happy, what I was dealing with in my life. ME.

But I'm not just me. I am a mother of three wonderful children. I am a wife. I am a daughter, a sister, an aunt, a godmother, and a friend. People count on me. With a clear brain, not all clouded up with alcohol, I know now that my children deserve a mother who is there for them. My husband deserves a wife who is present. And friends who have cared for me deserve the same in return. They will have their times when they need support, just as I have. My children will hear the news and be afraid, curious, worried, and confused. I am the one who is supposed to comfort them and protect them. I can only try to take that confusion and fear and try to turn it into solace and hopefully life lessons that will help them. There will always be bad news. Thanks to a wonderful friend, I am learning to look for the silver linings.

"Even the darkest night will end and the sun will rise."
– Victor Hugo

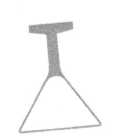

WAR OF MY WORLDS

On October 30, 1938, Orson Welles narrated the famous Halloween episode of *The Mercury Theater on the Air* radio drama anthology series that would go down in history. That episode's broadcast featured an adaptation of H.G. Wells' *The War of the Worlds*, creating widespread panic due to the radio reports of an alien invasion by Martians. In 1997, director Barry Levinson played on this theme in the film *Wag the Dog*, in which a fictitious war is created by a political campaign spin-doctor and a Hollywood producer in order to divert attention from a presidential sex scandal.

Now take that down about a million notches...here's my own little *War of the Worlds*. A purely selfish piece for me to turn to whenever I may get that strong urge to drink. What has helped me the most when I have a really overpowering craving is when someone tells me to "think it all the way through." In other words, don't just stop at the thought of how much you want a drink, and how good it would taste and feel, but continue the thought process all the way through to what happens AFTER.

Hopefully you won't skip this introduction and think this is real post about me picking up again...or I'll have a lot of 'splainin' to do! *The Walking Dead, Friday the 13th,* even *The Exorcist* do nothing to me compared to this—this scares the crap out of me. It doesn't have to be drinking or alcohol addiction, it can be whatever temptation you face that you know you have to fight. When your defenses get down and that little devil (temptation) on one shoulder is beating the crap out of the angel (conscience) on the other shoulder, think it through to the end.

Thanks for tuning in and letting me "think it through" here:

I guess it was a matter of time. I could only fight for so long. Salivating at the sight, or even thought, of a tall, smooth glass of wine. I picked up the drink, put the glass to my lips, closed my eyes and tilted it back. It was like a long lost friend giving me a huge hug. It warmed my entire body as it went down my throat, into my stomach and sent little sparks up to my brain. It was a feeling I hadn't experienced in such a long time. Almost two and a half years. A huge wave of thoughts came rushing back. First sip—check. Second sip here we go. This one was a little bigger, and faster. More warmth. More thoughts. And we're off to the races.

The glass was empty before I knew it. And I was feeling good again. That happy, euphoric feeling was coming back, pushing reality back down deep inside. The depression and anxiety were dissipating. The bottle wasn't far away—it was almost like a reflex that I always kept it close to my glass. I refilled my glass and put the bottle down, close again. As I sat and drank more, cares were rapidly thrown to the wind. This is totally fine, I thought. I got this. I can drink now and stop when I should, when I've had enough. It will be a one-time thing. Perhaps I could just return to my current path of sobriety and no one would know. I don't want to throw away all the time, days and chips I have accumulated. I don't want to have to change my sobriety date. No one will know. Fill 'er up again. And on it went, until the bottle was empty.

I felt great. More alive, carefree, and happy. Since I'm already drinking, just this one time, I may as well keep going. All in, if I'm going to be in at all. I look for another bottle. Not my preference, but it will do. It's got alcohol in it, which is really the only requirement at this point. I put on some music and sing along. Oh, how I missed this feeling. Better get something to eat. That's a smart plan. That will keep the alcohol from affecting me too much. Look, I'm even making sound decisions and using good judgement. That and the fact that I have the munchies.

But just then I hear the garage door. Crap. I can't let my family see that I've been drinking. I hide the empty bottle at the bottom of the trash can. I hide the open bottle, still half-full, behind a cabinet in the living room. As usual, I can't conceive of letting any of that precious liquid go to waste. A swift cleanup of the crime scene, a skill I had nearly perfected over the years. I quickly opened the peanut butter jar, swirled my finger in it and then rubbed it on my tongue. That should do the trick to hide the smell of the wine. I look in the mirror and rub the redness from the wine off my lips. Turn the music down. Grab my laptop. Just a normal night.

I listen to my children's updates from the day – school, sports, activities etc. I listen but I don't hear anything because the entire time my brain is preoccupied with trying to make sure I didn't leave out any incriminating evidence and that I don't appear at all tipsy. I go overboard trying to seem like super mom who is engaged and listening. Yet I have no idea what they are talking about.

My husband kisses me and I'm praying that all he can smell/taste is the peanut butter. He looks at me and I start to panic, wondering if he can tell. Or am I just being paranoid? He heads to our room to change, not appearing to suspect anything. But I turn around and see my daughter. She's looking at me with her beautiful blue eyes and seems to be looking right through me. Nah, she can't tell anything. She's *only thirteen. I ask her a few questions about her day, being careful to enunciate every word and not slur. I'm confident that I sound totally fine. I guess just as confident as I was all those other times. She heads off quietly to get ready for bed.*

I think about staying up and finishing the open bottle when they are all asleep. I hate to waste it. And I would have to get rid of it somehow anyway. But I'm starting to feel pretty light-headed. And tired. And drunk. It was just because I didn't eat, I'm sure. Brush my teeth and hit my pillow and I'm guessing I was out cold in a matter of seconds.

I woke up to the sound of one of my boys slamming the toilet seat down in the bathroom down the hall. I open one eye and quickly close it after it is attacked by beams of light breaking through the wood shutters. My head is pounding. Why? My mouth is dry and feels like a cat crawled in during the night and camped out on my tongue. Oh, shit. I have that horrible feeling I haven't had in quite a while—the confusion and fear over trying to remember why I felt the way I did. Hungover. No, it can't be. Let me think...ouch that hurts. Think more gently. Grab some water on my nightstand. As I guzzle it down, memories of gulping down wine last night start to emerge. Holy crap. There's no way I did that. Why? How am I going to face my family? I tell myself that they don't know. How could they? And how could I feel so hungover after only a bottle and a half of wine? It used to take much more than that.

I get up to go to the bathroom and my head pounds with each step. I'm feeling pretty nauseous now too, thinking that a tall glass of Coke on ice would hit the spot. When I make it to the bathroom, I get a glimpse of myself in the mirror. It's not pretty. A glimpse is all I can handle because I realize that there's no way I can look myself in the eyes. No one else may know. But I do. And no one else could possibly make me feel worse than I feel about myself right now.

I should get some coffee but I don't think I could stomach that. I need a Coke. But we never have any in our house. And that would be a dead giveaway as it was always my hangover drink of choice. Maybe a few crackers. Or a banana. Or stick my head in the freezer for a few seconds. All those things rushed into my brain, like instinct from the old days. I start to realize the significance of what I had done. All those battles I fought and won, only to lose the war by picking up a drink this one time.

How am I going to face anyone? My family? My friends from the program? My friends who have supported me? My friend who hasn't missed a day of checking in on me? My therapist? My blog readers? Myself? Shit. All that hard work just went down the toilet, along with the spit that was building up in my mouth as I got more nauseous. Almost 900 days. Ruined by one. Actually a few hours. Now my confusion started making its way to anger, then to guilt and on to shame. What have I done?

I have activated that ever-present, cunning, baffling and powerful disease inside. It is strong. It is clever. It is victorious. Game over. I lose. The dead guy in the hockey mask has caught me. The zombies have me cornered. My head is still spinning around in a complete circle despite the attempted exorcism. And I have become just another one of the high percentage of alcoholics who have relapsed. One publication from the National Institute on Alcohol Abuse and Alcoholism states that approximately 90 percent of alcoholics will experience one or more relapses during the four years after treatment. Other studies have relapse rates that range between 50–80%, and some say only one alcoholic out of three will be able to maintain sobriety. These are not very good odds. And they are very, very scary.

I always believed I was special. An exception. That I could beat the odds.

And now, I can either hang my head in shame and continue down a path that will eventually kill me, or I can pray for forgiveness and strength and get back on the right track to sobriety and what, I know for a fact, is a much better life.

I DID NOT DRINK. The above is all fictitious, and about me "thinking it through," perhaps a bit too realistically, since many people thought this was me talking about actually picking up. Real fear for me is not of Martians invading or the zombie apocalypse. It is fear of failing, i.e. going back to drinking.

My desire to succeed in staying sober is greater than my fear of failure right now. I will NOT pick up a drink. I don't want to feel like I imagined I would and described above. So Drink Devil on my shoulder, take a hike.

> *"Our greatest glory is not in never falling,*
> *but in rising every time we fall."*
> – **Confucius**

IF I CAN MAKE IT THERE...
I'LL MAKE IT ANYWHERE

This weekend, I sat in a beautiful apartment in NYC and looked out at an incredible view of the Statue of Liberty. The sun was shining and the sky was a slightly lighter shade of blue than the calm water. The serenity was such a sharp contrast to the feelings and energy surrounding my visit to this same city 2½ years ago. New York is the last place I had a drink of alcohol. Well, not just a drink but dozens of drinks. And the irony of the crisp, clear, cold, sunny day I took in with great clarity did not escape me. I don't remember what the weather was like when I woke up here in May of 2012, but I do remember that it wouldn't have mattered or had any effect on the foggy, grey and dark cloud that enveloped me.

I think it is safe to say that I have grown more and learned more in the past two and a half years than I have in all my other years prior. It's amazing what sobriety gives you. The gifts are too many to even list, but one of the biggest is time. Instead of your life passing you by in one big blur, you get to actually LIVE every day and be a part of your own life. Yes, there are days that are hard. Everyone has those. But to be able to feel those and actively participate in them is a gift as well.

Before one of my first sober solo adventures, a trip to meet a friend and go skiing in Colorado, I remember worrying about what I would do on a trip if I didn't drink. My travels always involved cocktails at whatever restaurants and bars we explored, cocktails while getting dressed to go out, cocktails after skiing, cocktails on the golf course, cocktails while dancing or listening to music, well, you get the idea. Going to a different city, state, country, whatever, always entailed researching what local culture we should experience. As I looked up restaurant reviews for the places I would be visiting, I noticed how many of them boasted about their specialty cocktails or extensive wine lists. And I started to sweat.

It turned out that I didn't have to waste one droplet of perspiration. There was plenty to do that didn't involve drinking. And guess what? It IS possible to enjoy great restaurants and bars—coffee bars maybe—and other places without cocktails. And even more enjoyable to wake up in the morning without a massive hangover. It's amazing what you can do when you don't feel like total crap.

On that 2012 trip to NYC, I almost didn't make it to the Broadway show we had tickets to because I was so miserably hungover I thought I was going to throw up. I don't remember any of the food we ate those few days because it was drowned out by all the cocktails and wine. I felt like crap, looked like crap and was probably pretty crappy company when I was hungover and shaking, in need of a drink.

On this trip to NYC, I enjoyed every minute of the three Broadway shows we saw. I savored every single morsel of food at great restaurants. I slept like a rock and woke up clear-headed and able to appreciate the beautiful view of the river and Lady Liberty. Conversations with my friend actually made sense (for the most part) and will be remembered. And, hopefully, I wasn't crappy company.

Sure, there were a few times I looked longingly at the cocktails that people at nearby tables were enjoying. And yes, I'd be lying if I said the bottle of vodka in the freezer and wine in the kitchen of the friend's apartment we stayed at didn't slightly temp me. But, as Ol' Blue Eyes sang, I wanted to be a part of it, AND make a brand new start of it. I think I did just that.

IF WE DON'T, THEN WHO WILL?

For nearly 40 years, I have watched the same holiday special on television, *A Charlie Brown Christmas*. As a child, I would rush to take my bath or shower and get into my pajamas so I could wrap myself in a blanket on the couch and watch it. As a teenager, I watched it with the small kids I babysat while their parents were out at holiday parties. And now, as a parent, I watch it with my own children, cuddled up with me in their pajamas in my bed.

My son kept saying that he didn't like the show because everyone was always mean to Charlie Brown. Why is everyone so mean to Charlie Brown? Good question. I love how sensitive he is. I told him he needed to watch it through to the end. I still well up with tears when all the kids belt out (with their mouths open wider than soccer balls) "Hark the Herald Angels Sing" to Charlie Brown and wish him a Merry Christmas at the end after they fix up his sad little tree.

What struck me this year was the speech Linus gives on the stage explaining the true meaning of Christmas. He quotes Luke from the bible:

"And there were in the same country shepherds abiding in the field, keeping watch over their flock by night. And lo, the angel of the Lord came upon them, and the glory of the Lord shone round about them: and they were sore afraid. And the angel said unto them, 'Fear not: for behold, I bring unto you good tidings of great joy, which shall be to all people. For unto you is born this day in the City of David, a Savior, which is Christ the Lord.

"And this shall be a sign unto you; Ye shall find the babe wrapped in swaddling clothes, lying in a manger.' And suddenly there was with the angel a multitude of the heavenly host, praising God, and saying, 'Glory to God in the highest, and on earth peace, good will toward men.'"

I hate to say it, but I fear that it is only a matter of time before this show is pulled from network television because of this monologue and its mention of Christ the Lord and God. I know, the horror. That a children's show, crammed in between commercials brainwashing them with all kinds of toys they should add to their Christmas lists, would dare incorporate a Christian message. It saddens me to say that I have become so disheartened by the "political correctness" of today's society, that I now actually expect someone, or some group, to petition to ban such programs from broadcast television. A show that has been televised every year since it was created in 1965 by a brilliant man named Charles Schulz.

Interestingly enough, it turns out that network executives were, in fact, reluctant to include the scene of Linus explaining the story of the birth of Christ. Apparently Charles Schulz was adamant that the scene remain, and said "if we don't tell the true meaning of Christmas, who will?" Clearly he won out. The scene stayed.

These days, we worry so much about offending someone that we often compromise our beliefs and values. We are so hung up on being politically correct, we tend to even shy away from talking about, writing about, or creating anything that might be the slightest bit controversial. I wouldn't be surprised if a child was sent home (or expelled) from school if he or she showed up with a t-shirt featuring Linus and his Christmas monologue. "Glory to God in the highest, and on earth peace, good will toward men."

Hell no. Not acceptable. Too controversial. God. Peace. Good will. Men. I'm not sure we are still allowed to talk about these things today.

I have always loved Snoopy and the Peanuts gang. I have always had great admiration for Charles Schulz and his creative genius, as well as his humility. He had no qualms about explaining that Charlie Brown's character was very much like himself, shy and awkward. But learning that he was adamant about keeping this scene in the Christmas special made me even more of a fan. I have a good friend who often says "if not me, then who…." for difficult situations that arise which most people wouldn't want to deal with. Think, just for a second, about how often that saying taken to heart would be helpful. If I don't volunteer to help, then who will? If I don't talk to my kids about bullying, drugs, drinking, etc., then who will? If I don't stand up for my convictions, then who will? And, in my case, if I don't tell my story about how I deal with my alcoholism and try to help others, then who will? Would it be easier to keep it quiet and deal with it privately? Yes. Would it have been easier for Schulz to cave to the television executives and remove the scene? Yes.

When you get lost in the frenzy of the holidays, take a minute and look up the scene from A Charlie Brown Christmas and listen to Linus. It will help you remember what Christmas is really all about. And, I gotta say, watching the kids dance while Schroeder plays the piano is pretty hilarious.

"I never eat December snowflakes.
I always wait until January."
– **Lucy Van Pelt,** *A Charlie Brown Christmas*

WHY ASK WHY?

I have a friend whose father, a brilliant man and artist, drank himself to death. I have another friend whose husband got lost in his addiction and also lost his life far too young. I have another friend who not only suffered the loss of someone very close when they committed suicide after battling alcoholism and depression, but also lost a friend in a car accident, and was clinically dead herself for a short time, when the car she was in was hit by a drunk driver. My great grandfather drowned in a boating accident when he was drunk. I hear countless stories in meetings, day after day, night after night, of women and men who have no relationships with their children, or aren't allowed to see their own grandchildren, because of their alcoholism. Other stories of intelligent, educated, "normal" people who spent years living on the street or behind bars due to their drinking or other addictions. So many lives affected and forever changed because of someone else's addiction and disease. Like storms with paths that left utter destruction. But yet here I sit, and somehow I can actually write that I wish I could have a drink right now. Mind boggling. And it scares the crap out of me.

I know what can happen if I pick up a drink and go back down the horrendous path that I was on. There is a reason why people say "change I must or die I will." There is no happy ending to alcoholism. Ever. I know all that and still salivate at the sight of, or often merely just the idea of, a big glass of red wine. It is insanity at its best. To think for a single second that I could miraculously now control my drinking.

But this time of year there is alcohol all around and the little Drink Devil in my head is constantly being fed ammunition. Every holiday-cheer cocktail party fuels the fire. And I need to ask and be reminded why I can't drink.

I liken it to the stage that most toddlers go through which is commonly referred to as the "Why" stage. Their little minds start expanding and curiosity takes over. The period may be brief, but for at least some length of time they ask "why" after just about everything you say. Time for bed. Why? You have to eat your vegetables. Why? Don't poke your baby brother in the eye. Why? How about because if you don't stop asking why I'm going to lose my mind. Why?

Call it the circle of life, or the oval of crap, or whatever you want to call it, but sometimes in my recovery and sobriety, I feel like I am reverting back to the maturity level of a toddler. I want to ask why to everything, starting with why can't I have a drink? To which I get the answer, because you are an alcoholic. Ok, why? Because you have a disease. Why? Umm, could be partly genetic, partly mental, partly physical, circumstantial, connected to depression...Why? It is what it is. Why? Because sometimes it is what it is and it just plain sucks.

And, sometimes when toddlers don't get the answers they want when they ask "why?" they throw a tantrum and stomp their feet. Along with my whys often comes anger. It doesn't make sense to me and it isn't fair that other people can drink and I can't. Waaa—waaa—waaa. Some people simply do not understand alcoholism and have had no experience with it. They cannot fathom why someone just simply can't stop drinking when they see all the problems it is causing in their life. Just stop drinking. If only it were that simple.

I hope to never leave a path of destruction behind me and I hate that people that I care about are still struggling because of one that was left for them. Does it suck? Yes. Do I want to be able to join the holiday fun and raise a glass with my friends? Yes. But it won't be one glass. Why? Because I am an alcoholic. So the simple "just stop drinking" for me comes with a whole lot of effort. And sometimes I get tired and want to stomp my feet. But when I'm tired and make it to the end of the day, I can sigh and smile. Why? Because I made it through another day without picking up a drink. How? One day at a time.

"He who has a why can endure any how."
– **Nietzsche**

WE HAD IT ALL WRONG

A woman gave me a card with this on it at a meeting the other night. I don't know who wrote it, but it sums up alcoholism very well.

> We drank for happiness and became
> UNHAPPY.
>
> We drank for joy and became
> MISERABLE.
>
> We drank for sociability and became
> ARGUMENTATIVE.
>
> We drank for friendship and made
> ENEMIES.
>
> We drank for sophistication and became
> OBNOXIOUS.
>
> We drank for sleep and awakened
> UNRESTED.
>
> We drank for strength and felt
> WEAK.
>
> We drank "medicinally" and acquired
> HEALTH PROBLEMS.
>
> We drank for relaxation and got
> THE SHAKES.
>
> We drank for bravery and became
> AFRAID.

We drank for confidence and became
  DOUBTFUL.

We drank to make conversation easier and
  SLURRED OUR SPEECH.

We drank to feel heavenly and ended up feeling
  LIKE HELL.

We drank to forget and were forever
  HAUNTED.

We drank for freedom and became
  SLAVES.

We drank to erase problems and saw them
  MULTIPLY.

We drank to cope with life and
  INVITED DEATH.

"It's not a person's mistakes that define them –
it's the way they make amends."
  – Freya North, *Chances*

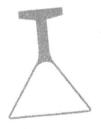

A SKEWED (OR SCREWED) POINT OF VIEW

People often say that we should try walking in someone else's shoes. Or they will tell us to try to see things from their point of view. We may hear "if I were you, I'd..." But you're not me. And I could put on your shoes and, whether they fit or not, the path I take is still my own. I can try out your glasses, even if they are rose-colored, and still not see things from your point of view. When we get lost in ourselves, or try to be someone or something we aren't, it helps to take a step back and try to find a way out. If we can't, we need to throw out a lifeline. It's who is there to catch it and reel you back in that matters. You need someone real to reel you in.

It's human nature to be self-centered to some point. We have to. Ultimately the only person who can take care of us is us. There are varying degrees of how much people put themselves first and how crucial they believe it to be. There are those who will tell you it's a dog-eat-dog world. Or every man for himself. Then, there are those who like to remind others that there is no 'I' in team-work. No man is an island. There are also people who constantly surround themselves with others but still feel incredibly lonely. Others like to be alone and are perfectly content to be their own best friend.

But back to being lost in ourselves. That can take us to a scary place. Our self-image is a conglomeration of judgments, feelings, thoughts, intuitions and ideas. Watch a baby when they first look into a mirror. They are completely fascinated. They will reach out to touch their new friend. Do they know it's them? I don't think so. They reach out and the image's hand reaches back. They knock their forehead up against the glass and their little friend does the same.

Now think about someone who has completely lost herself. I think at some point in life, we all look into a mirror and ask who the hell it is we are looking at. It's often surreal. It's the closest we can come to taking a step back and looking into our own life. We SEE what others see when they look at us. But we can feel something completely different. When we reach out our hand, there may be a deep-seated doubt, or fear, whether or not the other person in the mirror will in turn reach back to us.

We see a physical appearance that everyone else sees. But the feelings that the image churn up are unique to us. There are days when we look at that person with pride, and the shoulders go back a little more, the chin goes up, and the corners of the mouth turn upward in a complacent grin. Other days, we can look at that person with complete disgust, remorse, guilt and incredulousness that they did the things they did. Not us, but them.

We may attempt to splash cold water on our faces as if it could somehow change or clean up the image and the feelings associated with it. There was an old *Saturday Night Live* skit with Al Franken (now a United States Senator) as Stuart Smalley, where he would look into a mirror and tell himself aloud: "I'm good enough, I'm smart enough, and doggone it, people like me!" The segment was called "Daily Affirmations."

Sometimes, we do need to convince ourselves that what or who we see in the mirror is okay. A little pep talk. Being able to do this ourselves, self-affirmation, is a hugely important skill. For most of my life, I have been way too hung-up on what other people think of me. My need for external validation was surpassed only by my need for ice cream. Learning to rely more on myself and my own gut-check and less on the approval of others is a life-long lesson in growth.

Without a drink in my hand, the mirror becomes less cloudy. The Greek in me has used the Windex to wipe it clean, little by little. And I try to remember this:

"And here is my little secret, a very simple secret:
It is only with the heart that one can see rightly.
What is essential is invisible to the eye."
– Antoine de Saint-Exupéry, *The Little Prince*

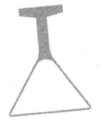

THE GHOST OF CHRISTMAS PAST

While writing my blog is immensely cathartic for me, my goal is to help other people struggling to overcome alcoholism. Not just alcoholism or addiction, but any demon that they face. As I work to stay one step ahead of mine and follow the path to a much happier, healthier life, I hope that sharing my stories will help others see that it's never too late to turn things around. Whatever adversity they face.

The holidays are a rough time for many people, including alcoholics. The parties, the expectations, the stress, the associations and memories. Year after year, I remember just sitting, in the dark, looking at our Christmas tree and its beautiful lights and ornaments, with several glasses of wine or cocktails du jour, and crying. Quietly crying. Why did such a beautiful symbol of Christmas always bring me so down? Or was I just down and the Christmas tree smacked me in the face to remind me? Depression is its own monster (though intricately connected to alcoholism). While we usually think of it as the blues, this time of year it just comes in red and green.

Past Christmases brought some wonderful memories back to me. There were several years when my brothers and I would hike through the woods behind my grandparents' house and pick out the perfect Christmas tree. My grandfather would chop it down with pride and carry it back down, through the snow, to our car. Often, the tree ended up looking quite like Charlie Brown's feeble little tree, but we always loved it nevertheless.

When we were kids, our dear family friends, who were Jewish, would come decorate our tree with us. In turn, they invited us to celebrate a night of Hanukah with them and taught us about lighting the menorah and their traditions. It was a wonderful way to experience the holidays together. Not to mention the incredible potato latkes and matzah brie we got to eat! (Thank you Aunt B.!)

But this year, when the house was quiet and the kids were asleep, I was able to sit and look at our beautiful tree, and smile. It was decorated by my children. And it was a happy symbol to me. No wine. No cocktails. No tears. Believe me, there were times very recently when I thought I was losing the battle and that the Drink Devil was pouring a glass for me. Get lost. 31 months yesterday without a single drop. Take that.

I don't do it on my own, however. I can't. My battle gear is multi-layered. First and foremost, I send my HP (Higher Power) in first. Going to meetings stores up the ammo I need to fight. And my family and friends back me up and provide me with additional armor. Thank you doesn't really cut it, but until I find better words, that's all I can say. Thank you, each and every one of you, for your support and encouragement. All while you have your own battles to fight. I don't think that you have any idea how much just a small gesture means—a hug, a kind word, a pat on the back, a "like" or a "share" of my work, or even taking the time to explain to me what I could do better. Short emails that say "you rock" make my day. You are the one who rocks for taking the time to send that.

As I have said before, I realize that everyone has their own cross to bear. Most people fight their battles quietly and bravely in their own way. I have chosen to share mine openly and publicly, which I understand not everyone will agree with. I get my share of criticism with my writing as well. I have to learn to take the good with the bad. But, the number of people who have written to me or told me how much a piece I wrote helped them makes it all worth it. Kneeling on the floor, throwing up in the toilet, head pounding, hungover, humiliated and ashamed, is a scenario I don't wish to repeat and I don't wish upon anyone else.

I'd be right back there if the Drink Devil wins. My writing helps get those bad thoughts out of my head and takes away most of their power. I hope somehow it helps you too.

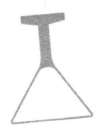

SHARING THE LIGHT

"And when you want to live, how do you start,
where do you go, who do you need to know?"
— The Smiths, "The Boy with the Thorn in His Side."

As you may have noticed by now, I'm very fond of quotes. I usually include at least one with every blog piece I write. My philosophy is: why not share the brilliant words of others instead of struggling to find a way to say it (less eloquently) myself? I also like to call it "sharing the light." Some of the best quotes and pearls of wisdom I hear are in meetings. And many of them are said by people who are quoting someone else, or sharing the light. Sometimes I hear the same platitude or trite saying again and again, but for some reason, one particular time, it finally gets through my thick skull. For alcoholics, there are many. But as you can see, they can apply to a myriad of situations, self-helpers and, especially, serenity seekers:

One day at a time

Let go and let God

Change I must or die I will

Do the next right thing

But for the grace of God

The best is yet to come

Turn it over

Keep an attitude of gratitude

Get rid of the stinkin' thinkin'

But the best by far is the Serenity Prayer. If we can just remember that, things would be much easier. For everyone. Not just alcoholics or addicts. Everyone. When times are tough and things aren't going your way, simply remember this:

"God, grant me the serenity
To accept the things I cannot change,
The courage to change the things I can,
And the wisdom to know the difference."

Really think about that. If we learn to accept the things we cannot change, we would take away a huge chunk of unnecessary worry and stress. Courage is something we could all use, especially courage to take control of situations where we have the ability to make things better. And wisdom, well, that goes without saying. But wisdom to know the difference isn't always easy to come by.

Working toward sobriety and a better life, and changing old destructive ways, IS something I have the ability to control. The disease of alcoholism I cannot change. It's there. I didn't ask for it but it's there. And it's there for good. I accept that. The courage to change how I deal with it and fight it is something I continue to pray for. The wisdom to know the difference comes from those who share the light with me, and of course, from my Higher Power (HP).

As for my Smiths quote, "when you want to live, how do you start, where do you go, who do you need to know?"—I loved the Smiths in high school and college. I still do. Many of Morrissey's morbid and depressing lyrics used to blast from my car radio. They fit in perfectly with my teenage angst and misery of the time. But the quote above always gave me hope. I think it is honestly something that I asked myself deep down many times when I was struggling to crawl out of the terrible dark hole I was in.

Now that I have the clarity of my sobriety, I can answer those questions. When you want to live, you start by simply making that choice. That you want to LIVE. In a twelve-step program, that's always the first step. Where do you go and who do you need to know? Also simple. You need to know where to find those who share the light with you and those who care. You need to know and establish a strong connection to your HP. You need to remember the serenity prayer. And, that some girls are bigger than others... (Smiths).

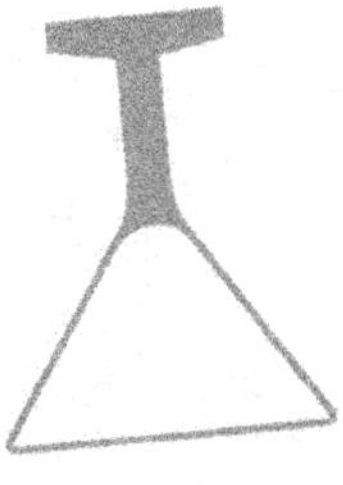

NAMASTE

I went to yoga yesterday for the first time in quite a while. I haven't been able to go because I broke my collarbone badly. How? Falling off a motorcycle. And in full disclosure, it wasn't even moving. Yup, ambulance ride and all. Five days in the hospital. Surgery. And pain meds. The E.R. doctors immediately started pumping me with morphine to handle the pain. And I immediately started telling them that I am a recovering alcoholic. I've heard too many stories about cross-addiction to take any chances. I wanted to get off the pain medication as soon as I possibly could. My husband kept track of them for me and doled them out on a strict schedule.

But back to the accident. Who falls off a stationary motorcycle? That takes real talent. Thank you very much. Then again, I also allowed a ladder to swing down from our attic and hit me smack in the face, giving me a nasty concussion and stitches right between my eyes.

What's even more pathetic is that I was completely SOBER for both of these accidents. In fact, I've done more bodily harm to myself sober than I did when I was drinking (not counting the hideous toll the alcohol took on the inside of my entire body). How is that possible? When I drank, I know I fell down countless times. I also know that one night, I went tumbling down a very steep staircase, which honestly could have killed me. Somehow, ironically, we become invincible (or so we think) when we drink.

I figured yoga would be relatively low risk for me to injure myself. Then again, if anyone could turn yoga into a dangerous, contact sport it would be me. Instead of some graceful swan pose,

I'd be more likely to transition into falling crane, losing my balance and tumbling into the person next to me. I love yoga but it requires me to be still and sit quietly with myself, something I am not very good at. The teacher instructs us to allow thoughts to come into our mind, acknowledge them and then immediately dismiss them. If I could control my mind like that, I'd be pulling some Uri Geller moves and bending spoons or doing the laundry just by thinking about it. It actually takes practice to be able to sit still and be quiet inside yourself. I need way more practice.

While I get into warrior pose, I start going through my grocery list in my head. And then I look at the cool yoga pants on the woman next to me and think to myself that I should get some like that. I wonder where she got them. Oops we have moved on to the next pose, which requires balance. Time for me to hit child's pose. I'll stay here for a while. And try to remember what kinds of ice cream I have in the freezer or if I have to go get some on the way home from yoga. As you can tell, I clearly need more practice at quieting my mind.

There were days early on in my sobriety when I tried to do yoga and after about ten minutes, I just slumped into child's pose and wanted to give up. I was tired, weak, miserable and sometimes still shaking. I also liked to lie flat on my back and call it corpse pose. Luckily, the yoga teacher was very understanding and simply asked if I was ok. I hope what will come with the practice will be longer periods of time where I can be still and just be.

If I can take this practice with me out into the real world, perhaps I can even learn to simply acknowledge the thought of wanting a drink and then let it go. Right now, that thought sometimes comes and sets up camp in my brain and won't leave. Like last night and tonight. It would have been nice if the concussion could have somehow knocked that part of my brain out too.

The quiet, reflective time is not just a suggested practice but is actually an active part of recovery. Meditation and prayer work wonders. As I've said many times before, I have to constantly remind myself of the serenity prayer as well as of the need to turn things over to my HP.

When my mind is quiet and I can be still, I can remember to do those things. If you haven't tried yoga, I highly recommend it. And if you see someone in the back of the room wearing a helmet and spending most of the class in child's pose, that's me.

"To the mind that is still, the whole universe surrenders."
– Lao Tzu

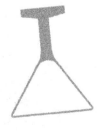

HOME OF THE BRAVE

I went to a meeting today because I started to feel a craving coming on. I stopped on the way at 7-11 to get candy, thinking it might help as a substitute for alcohol and fulfill my sugar craving. I'm learning that when I really want to get to a meeting, it means I really need one. A young guy led the meeting and told his story. Really tough to listen to. He said he joined the Army with his best friend when he was 18. They served in Iraq together and on two occasions, his best friend saved his life. On the second, he was killed while doing so. He continued to share about being wounded and hospitalized, and also how he suffered from PTSD. I hear so many horrible stories in meetings but this one really got to me. He had only 52 days of sobriety but had such a positive attitude and determination that I know that his count will continue to go up.

People tell me that they can't imagine how hard it is for me not to drink. They say they admire my courage in sharing my story so that it might help others. What I do is nothing compared to this man. That's real courage. To go through and witness the horror he did and be determined to get himself healthy again. That's bravery. To build up his strength to fight a disease that tempts him constantly by providing a temporary respite from the torturous images in his mind. Heroic. My guess is that his determination comes from knowing that his best friend didn't save his life and lose his own so he could kill himself with alcohol. He killed many enemy combatants on his tour, but the toughest, strongest one he has to battle is inside himself.

I often think about whether or not I would be strong enough to maintain my sobriety if something traumatic happened. In an earlier piece I wrote, called "Weak Enough," I talked about the need not to be strong enough, but to be weak enough to turn it over to God. Of course I hope nothing traumatic happens, but to show how twisted an alcoholic's thinking can be, another man at the meeting said that sometimes he fantasizes about something tragic happening so he would have an excuse to drink. Think about that. Wanting something bad to happen to give you an "excuse" to reunite with your old friend the bottle.

That's why I go to meetings. Every meeting is like putting a deposit in the sobriety bank so that when the shit really hits the fan, I will have plenty in there to withdraw. Maybe this young, newly sober soldier sees meetings as ammo that he stores up for himself, and extracting from that cache when he needs to fight that vicious enemy inside. You have to do whatever it is that works for you to fight the battle with a disease that is cunning, baffling and powerful.

For this young man, and for all like him who served our country, thank you for your service. And thank you for thinking enough of yourself, and your best friend, to make this life the best you can, one day at a time.

> *"Gold is good in its place, but living, brave,*
> *patriotic men are better than gold."*
> – Abraham Lincoln

I SEE A SHIP IN THE HARBOR

As awful and difficult as they can be, funerals provide an opportunity to reflect, take a look at your own life and reassess the path you are taking. I went to a funeral yesterday for a wonderful woman I met during my recovery. She took me with her to speak to a group of women at the local detention facility. She had been going faithfully to meet with women in jail for over twenty years. That was just one group she reached out to help.

On the evening we rode to the jail together, she shared with me some of her amazing story. She had lived a fascinating life as a journalist and traveled all over the world. She worked for various organizations and associations that helped women around the globe. I could have listened to her stories for hours, and hoped to have more opportunities to do so. But I won't. I told her she should really write a book. But she won't.

Her husband spoke at the funeral and gave a detailed biography and list of selfless achievements. He said that the thing she was most proud of, of all these things, was her sobriety date. She considered it the day that God removed from her the compulsion to drink. September 21, 1981. Not a drink since then. He shared with the small group gathered to pay their respects that she did not want to just experience this wonderful, new, sober, improved life alone, but wanted to share it with others. So she reached out wherever she could and was a mentor and support to many people, mostly women, along her path through sobriety.

A young rabbi presided over the funeral and recounted a well-known and comforting story based on a quote from Ecclesiastes 7:1: "The day of death is better than the day of one's birth." He explained that when a person is born, people rejoice and when one dies, everyone cries. That, he told us, is backwards. He said that when a person is born, everyone should cry because there is no way of knowing whether he or she will follow the right path in their life. When a person dies, however, everyone should celebrate since they know that he or she left this world in peace after living a good life on the correct path, like my friend.

The rabbi went on to say that this story can be compared to two ships that were in the water, full of cargo. One ship was coming in to port and the other was leaving. People were focused on and praising the ship coming into port, and not the one going out on its new adventure. Why? Because the incoming ship had departed in peace and arrived at its destination in peace. But no one knows what the future holds for the ship that is just beginning its journey. "So it is with a person who is born: we do not know the nature of his future deeds. But when he leaves this world, we know the nature of his deeds." *(Yalkut Shimoni Kohelet 7:1.)*

The Beth El Synagogue Center website sums this up beautifully:

"This tale knows that we cry when someone we love passes. At the same time, it asks that we focus on how the person lived, rather than on a death that comes to us all. It values the deeds the person engaged in, and views the totality of human life as a lesson from which we can learn; and it does so with a sense of humility. We cannot know with certainty what life holds in store for us, nor what awaits us after we die, even though Judaism believes in an afterlife of the soul. But we can choose to live with God and with righteousness regardless of what storms come our way."

As sad as it was to lose someone wonderful, I was comforted by this service. It did indeed focus on how she lived a life on the right path and with great humility. Something to think about and hopefully learn from. On the way out of the funeral, another friend from recovery took hold of my arm to walk out together.

She asked me if I thought that the other people there knew who we were—the group of recovering alcoholic women who sat together and came to pay respects to their friend. I told her that I was pretty sure they did, and that I was proud of that.

On September 21, I'll have a pint of *Ben and Jerry's* out, with 2 spoons, to toast my friend's sobriety date and the wonderful woman that she was.

"On the death of a friend, we should consider that the fates through confidence have devolved on us the task of a double living, that we have henceforth to fulfill the promise of our friend's life also, in our own, to the world."
– Henry David Thoreau

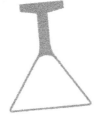

WHEN THE PASTOR NEEDS A PRAYER...
AND THE DOCTOR NEEDS THE CARE

There's a guy who is often seen running around here, bandana on his head, beard keeping his face warm and boyish countenance looking a little older, and short shorts showing off his runner's legs. If you didn't know who he was, you might be a little surprised to learn that he is a pastor. Not just a pastor, but a darn good one. And he's not even my pastor, but I'm honored to call him a friend. He's also one of the smartest people you will ever meet. And one of the most humble. He's a father, a husband, a leader of mission trips to other parts of the world and an incredible writer/blogger. He's a source of comfort to so many in our community and even around the world. And now, he has cancer. While I usually don't consider myself at a loss for words, all that comes to mind now is that it sucks. Plain and simple. It sucks.

I wrote a guest blog piece for him a while back called "Consider It Pure Joy," about the book of James. I quoted the opening lines of that book of the Bible: "Consider it pure joy, my brothers and sisters, whenever you face trials of many kinds because you know that the testing of your faith produces perseverance."

My lay translation of that was this: Be glad that you are going through living hell right now because it will make you stronger. At the time, I was linking this passage in James with my alcoholism. Somehow I don't think this young pastor or his family are considering any of this joy or feel the slightest bit of gladness right now.

So what happens when the one who gives the prayers needs the prayers? I have no doubt that he will have many, many prayers heading his way. They have already started rolling in (or up). I am reminded of a similar situation when it was the doctor who needed the care. My father, who helped so many people over the span of decades as an excellent urologist and skilled surgeon, suffered a stroke himself just six months after he retired. A man who never smoked, hardly drank at all, was meticulous about what he ate and exercised regularly. I guess in many cases, if it's in your genes, well, you're screwed. A little like alcoholism. But my friend's cancer? Don't think so. He is another guy who takes excellent care of his body and mind.

My father learned what it was like to be the one lying in the bed being cared for and waiting anxiously for the doctor's updates instead of being the one giving them. He was quoted in an article that was written about him called "When the Doctor Becomes the Patient" as saying that he thought every physician should spend some time on the other side (or in the bed) to gain an appreciation for what the patient goes through and experiences. He gained a new appreciation for the nurses, staff and physical therapists who helped him back on his feet, literally, as he was paralyzed on his right side by the stroke.

But what about the pastor? Is this the other side for him? Being the one needing to receive the prayers and blessings instead of being the one to administer them? He just wrote a blog piece himself that said "not only is my faith expected to be a resource for me while cancer tries to kill me, it's expected my faith vs. the cancer will be a resource to others too." Yes, high expectations when you are public with your struggle. But you can see his thoughts are already turned to others in this tough time.

I wrote another piece recently called "Why Ask Why?" In this situation? Who the hell knows why. It doesn't make any sense. But we are supposed to believe that there is a reason and that God has this all in his plans. We may not understand the plans and certainly don't have to like them. But somehow we have to keep the faith. Don't ask me why. I would ask Him.

> *"Never be afraid to trust an unknown future to a known God."*
> – **Corrie ten Boom**

ONE THOUSAND SHADES OF SOBER

Today marks the 1000th day of my sobriety. 1000 freaking days without a single drop of booze. Gotta say I'm pretty amazed by that myself. There were so many days and nights when I thought I would cave. But I didn't. So what did I decide to do? Celebrate. Yep, I threw myself a big ol' par-tay. A mocktail party. With all the people who have supported me and been there for me when I needed help. People who took time out of their busy lives to send me a quick text or email or share a few words of encouragement. In this case, though, I wasn't sure that if I built it they would come. But they did. Through a miserable snow/sleet/freezing rain storm on a frigid night. They came out, despite those conditions, and no booze, to celebrate with me. I was truly overwhelmed.

Like I said, I had my doubts about throwing this party. Would people want to go to a party on a Saturday night with no alcohol? For a few, the answer was no. For many, the answer was hell yes. I'm sure the fact that we have all been cooped up in our houses with our kids due to the weather added to everyone's enthusiasm for a night out. The invitation asked that guests bring a creative, non-alcoholic drink and that prizes would be awarded for Best Tasting Mocktail and Best Mocktail Name. There were some REALLY creative names and drinks. A few favorites were: "Abstinence on the Beach," "Sans-gria," "No Way Jose Mango-rita," "Berry-Lime Hickey," and 'You Bet Your Blueberry Ass!" But the most votes went to "Still Have My Hymen Sangria." Pretty funny. People seemed to have a fun time tasting and voting for their favorites.

In addition to the mocktail mania, we had a "Candy Bar" with all my favorite sugary treats. A few sugar hangovers today, but I'll take that any day over the old days of puking and spending the entire day after in bed. It was definitely more fun than I had even imagined and, for the first time in a long time, I enjoyed a party and wasn't drooling over the wine I couldn't drink or searching for the door to plan my exit. We built it. They came. And it meant a great deal to me. One friend said as she was leaving, "You know, no one came for the food, or for the drinks, or to have a night out. They came for you. To celebrate your amazing achievement." What does one say to that?

I am happy that my kids were there helping and mingling so that they could see adults having a great time WITHOUT any alcohol. I am happy that I was able to have coherent conversations that I actually remember. I am happy that we all woke up feeling refreshed and not hungover. I am happy that people came and enjoyed themselves on a nasty, wintery night. I hope that everyone who came, and those who couldn't, know how much I appreciate their kindness and support. God willing, they will be there with me to celebrate 2000 days. When I get the urge to pick up a drink, I can think of that and continue to fight even harder. There's a whole world out there that can be just as fun, if not more so, sober.

"Happiness lies in the joy of achievement
and the thrill of creative effort."
– Franklin Roosevelt

"If you build it, they will come."
– Theodore Roosevelt

LIFE IS ALL ABOUT ME

Those who know me well know that I constantly joke that life is all about me. In keeping with that tenet, I brought up the subject of selfishness at a meeting the other day. Does putting my sobriety first make me a selfish person? I was reminded that when we travel on a plane, the flight attendants always tell us during the safety demonstrations to put our own oxygen masks on first and then help our children or anyone else who may need assistance. We must first take care of ourselves so we can take care of others. Without oxygen to breathe, we won't be able to help anyone.

In my world, without my sobriety, I can't be of any use to anyone else, especially my children. Without my sobriety, I'm not there for them. I'm not even there for me. When I drank, however, it really was all about me. And my drinks. And my time to drink. And my deserving to drink. So am I selfish now when I put sobriety first? I don't think so. Without my sobriety, I slip back into a dark place—a hole that I would have to struggle to get out of.

By putting sobriety first, I mean that it is my first priority, every day. I have a friend who says she starts every day with her own "happy hour"—some quiet time of prayer and meditation. Many in recovery know that SLIP stands for "Sobriety Lost Its Priority."

There were too many really bad "selfs" while we were in the midst of our drinking—self-doubt, self-loathing, low self-esteem, no self-confidence and very little self-worth. The selfish drinking washed those all away, for a little while at least. But in the numbing, dull ache that came with inebriation, I lost my "self."

As hard as I work my program of recovery, a whole lifetime set in self-centeredness cannot be reversed all at once. But on this journey into sobriety, I have found a whole new world of "selfs"— self-awareness, self-discovery, self-respect, self-preservation. A twelve-step program has very little room for ego. In fact, in step three, we "made a decision to turn our will and our lives over to the care of God as we understood Him." Self-will is traded in for God's will. Ego is thrown out the window.

When we get to the twelfth step, we encounter the dichotomy of helping others after all the time spent on helping ourselves. The truth, however, is that in helping others, we are in fact helping ourselves. Our selflessness is actually to our own benefit. Back to our selfishness as a recovering alcoholic. I find that the following quote from the Dalai Lama explains this best:

> "It is important that when pursuing our own self-interest we should be 'wise selfish' and not 'foolish selfish.' Being foolish selfish means pursuing our own interests in a narrow, shortsighted way. Being wise selfish means taking a broader view and recognizing that our own long-term individual interest lies in the welfare of everyone. Being wise selfish means being compassionate."

I hope that I fall into the category of "wise selfish" and compassionate rather than foolish selfish. A few people have expressed their opinions that my life is too focused on my sobriety. That my recovery shouldn't define me. My past mistakes and addiction may not define me, but they made me who I am today. And after 1,005 days without a drink, I am pretty proud of who I am today.

SOBRIETY IN JEOPARDY

"Sometimes sobriety sucks."

Please remember to respond in the form of a question.

Oh, ok. "What is sometimes sobriety sucks?"

I'll take "Everyday Battles" for $400 please, Alex.

Answer: "This term is used to describe 5pm on Friday."

Question: "What is Suckfest?"

You are correct.

Let's take a moment to meet our players. Joe Q. is a seventh grade history teacher from Springfield, Illinois. He's got an interesting story to tell us about his cats.

Yes, thanks, Alex. Well, one time, my cats, Sam and Mr. Mittens, were looking out the window and saw me coming home from work….

That's fascinating. On to our next contestant. Sarah W. Sarah, that's an interesting shawl you're wearing. Do you want to tell us about it?

No.

All righty then. Our final contestant, Mike S., is celebrating 25 years of sobriety. Can you tell us your secret to staying sober Mike?

Well, Alex, I refrain from drinking.

Excellent advice, Mike. Thanks for sharing.

Now back to the game. Mike, you control the board.

Actually Alex, I'm powerless over the board. I'm first-stepping the board.

What the hell does that mean Mike?

It means that I am admitting I am powerless over the board and that my life has become unmanageable because of the board.

Mike, we're talking about a game show here. You have control over what category you choose.

Do I really have control, Alex? Or do I just have a daily reprieve? Can I actually change the board? Do I have the courage to change the board? Remember, Alex: God, grant me the serenity to accept the things I cannot change, the courage to change the things I can, and the wisdom to know the difference.

OK, Mike, well, I have the wisdom to move on to Sarah. Sarah, please pick our next clue.

I'd like to buy a vowel.

Wrong game show, Sarah.

Oh sorry. I'll take "Codependency" for $600 please Alex.

Ok, here's our clue: "Pleasing others and giving up yourself."

I think that the answer is: "What is a sign of codependency?" Do you think so, Alex, I mean, I think that's what it is, if that's what you think it is. I'm not sure. But if you think I should guess that, then I will. Do you want me to guess that, Alex?

Correct. Pick again.

I'll take "Trite AA Slogans" for $800 please.

Ok. And that's a Daily Double. What would you like to do?

I'll make it a true Daily Double, Alex. I don't know what that really means, as opposed to a false Daily Double, but I always wanted to say it.

Um, great, Sarah. You're betting everything you have then. Ok. Here's the clue:

"This common AA saying rhymes with, 'Run Way Bat a Dime.'"

"What is First Thing's First?"

Um, No. Mike? Joe? ... Do either of you want to take a guess?

"What is Easy Does It?"

Holy cow, what is wrong with you people??? A saying that rhymes with "Run Way Bat a Dime?" *One Day At a Time*??? Sound familiar??

Don't judge, just love, Alex.

Let's go to a commercial break...so I can have a freaking drink.

"Our life is a game, the rules of which are unknown to us."
— Søren Kierkegaard

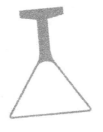

UNFAIR BECAUSE WE CARE

In a city like Washington, D.C., I've seen my share of good things happen to bad people. People getting ahead by lying, cheating and clawing their way to the top. Enough instances that make me want to declare that life isn't fair. But lately, I've been seeing way too many examples of bad things happening to good people. Things that make me want to shout at the top of my lungs that life is, indeed, not fair. I usually adhere to the belief that everything happens for a reason. That what goes around comes around. That God has a plan. Karma. But, for the life of me, I cannot understand how there could possibly be a reason for such bad things to happen to good people. Great people. Innocent people. Seemingly healthy people.

So I turned to the Bible to see what words of wisdom I could find. Proverbs 3:5-6 says "trust in the Lord with all your heart and lean not on your own understanding." Okay, that helps a little. I can't lean on my own understanding because I have no understanding here. How about Ephesians 6:11: "Put on the full armor of God so that you can take a stand against the devil's schemes." Ok. Put on the full armor of God. How do I do that? What if these good people took a stand against the devil's schemes and lost? I've quoted the book of James a few times in my blog posts, but these things hardly seem to qualify to fall under the category of "consider it pure joy... whenever you face trials of many kinds because you know that the testing of your faith produces perseverance." These people have faith. And they have perseverance. But there is no joy in the trials they are facing that I can see.

Then I found this quote: "Accepting that life is insane, that bad things happen to good people and that you can find the courage to be grateful for the good in every situation and still move forward is hard (even terrifying), but heroic." (Richie Norton, author and CEO of Global Consulting Circle). Given the current situations, I would agree that life is insane. I would also stand by my observation that life is not fair. I can worry. I can whine. I can wallow in the suckiness. I can try to fathom why some people get sick when they take really good care of themselves. None of that will help in the least. But I don't see how to "be grateful for the good" in these situations. They all lead back to the question of why?

I wrote an entire piece entitled "Why Ask Why?" and I still don't have any answers. Why? Because we have the need to try to understand. To try to make sense of things. But often we simply cannot. Why do we care? And why do we try to make sense out of things? Often the answer is simply this: we care because we love.

It's difficult, no, it's torturous, to watch the people we love suffer. In any way, shape or form. We wish we had the power to fix things for them, but we don't. We wish we could explain to them why, but we can't. We can scream at the top of our lungs that it's not fair, but will anyone hear? If they do hear, will they listen and help change it? We can raise our fist and look upward and ask how a peaceful, loving God could allow such things to happen. That's the big mystery. How and why?

But I have heard of and seen first-hand the power of prayer. Miraculous stories of healing and change brought about by faith and prayer. And I would rather love and feel the pain than not love at all. So the verse I'm going to stick with is this: 1 Corinthians 13:7-9 "Love bears all things, believes all things, hopes all things, endures all things. Love never fails."

"The world isn't fair, Calvin."
"I know Dad, but why isn't it ever unfair in my favor?"
– Bill Watterson, *Calvin and Hobbes*

SLOWLY I TURNED, STEP BY STEP...

I remember watching *"Abbott and Costello"* on the weekends with my brothers when we were kids. I still laugh when I think about the "Slowly I Turned..." vaudeville sketch they did. The routine features a man dramatically relating the tale of getting revenge on his enemy. He becomes so riled up in telling the story that he attacks the innocent listener (Costello). The man seems to regain his composure until someone once again says something that triggers another outburst and attack.

Strangely, this sums up how I feel about working my twelve steps in recovery. I make progress, step by step, and then WHAM! – something arms the cunning disease with more ammo to attack me. Especially when it comes to the fourth step. Step Four in the Twelve Step program in which I participate says we are to have "made a searching and fearless moral inventory of ourselves." Many of you know what I mean when I say this is much easier said than done. This is where we need to pull up our big girl panties (or big boy boxers) and take a serious look at our shortcomings and character defects, (which we humbly ask to be removed in Step Seven).

It's taken me nearly 35 months of sobriety to get to my fourth step. Well, actually, I've gotten to it. I just haven't gotten past it. So I sat down the other night and started writing. And writing. And going through my memories and writing more. Wow. Looking back at it now, I can't believe that I didn't see all the red flags about my alcoholism. Or even just a few of them. I guess it's true when they say you won't see it until you are ready.

I think everyone could benefit from doing the fourth step. A chance to take a look at the skeletons in one's closet, air them out, and then bury them for good. Alcoholic or not, everyone has regrets. Everyone has traits that they would like to improve upon or change. Some try to ignore the past. Some beat themselves up over it. Some carry the guilt, remorse and shame around with them as heavy baggage. The hard part comes from stepping up (ha) and finding the courage to actually make the change or unpack the baggage and put it down, once and for all. Step Four can take you down a dark and scary road. Coming out on the other side, into the sunlight, takes some hard work but it's well worth it.

I'm not saying that it's as easy as deciding to make the change and simply letting go of the burden of past mistakes. It's extremely difficult. As we look back, and take our "searching and fearless moral inventory," sometimes things bubble up to the surface from deep down that we had forgotten or subconsciously repressed. Layers of the onion begin to peel off. As open as I am with my struggle with alcoholism, in the hope that I can help others, there are things that I could never imagine sharing. But according to Step Five, we have to admit to "God, to ourselves, and to one other human being the exact nature of our wrongs." The one other human being can be anyone you choose—friend, sponsor, therapist, clergy, etc. No, the basketball that you draw a face on and call "Joe" doesn't count.

Unfortunately, Step Four can be too tough for many alcoholics or addicts to tackle. The skeletons in the closet are more like tenacious zombies that are not ready to be put to rest. And some don't understand that while God forgives their past regressions, they have to forgive themselves before they can move on. Later in the Twelve Steps, we come to the part where we have to make amends to those whom we have harmed. In many cases, some of these can not be made, whether it's because the person is no longer alive, unable to be reached, or when making the amends would "injure them or others".

I'm not proud of some of the things I've done. And looking back through years of therapy, I can see more clearly some of my character defects, especially the insecurity and low self-esteem, that led to much of the regretful behavior. But I feel that the best thing I can do, the most helpful "step" in the right direction, is to make a living amend. To make an attempt every day to do the next right thing and live my life in a way that atones for past mistakes. To be present with my kids and my husband, to be a better friend to those who bless me with their friendship and to make the choice every day to take the next step down the right path.

> *"We are products of our past, but we don't have to be prisoners of it."*
> – Rick Warren, *The Purpose Driven Life*

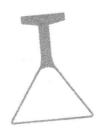

SUMMER IS AROUND THE CORNER

It's that time of year again. Time to sign kids up for summer camps. It's a love/hate thing. While I love the idea of the kids being at camps and not driving me insane 24/7, the logistics can be a nightmare. Sometimes I think I need an engineer from NASA to come draw me a schematic or flow chart of who is going where and when. And what happened to the good old days when our parents would kick us out in the morning and tell us to come home in time for dinner? A different world, that's for sure. What happened to kids using their imaginations and creating a space rocket out of an empty, giant cardboard box? Now they control a space rocket on the screen of some sort of an electronic gadget to destroy alien invaders or to build their own futuristic cities.

These days, if you don't send your kids to all kinds of different summer camps, it seems like they are left to fend for themselves, with few friends around to play with. God forbid they aren't entertained every second of the day. There is pretty much a camp for everything too—boy scout camp, art camp, basketball camp, yoga camp, junior architect camp, sumo wrestling camp... For some parents, camps aren't enough. They want their kids to be learning during the summer as well, so they register them for summer school or extra classes like Introduction to Swahili or Norse Mythology. Surely those will help Johnny get into Harvard. There are also numerous vacation Bible camps, and by August, I am honestly fine with enrolling them in Satanic Cult camp if it gets them out of my hair.

Then there are the carpools. With three kids going in three different directions, these can be more confusing than and about as fucked up as Obamacare. Take child 1 to pick up three of his friends and drop them at chess camp, child 2 is getting picked up by another mom to go to frog hunting camp, and child three is still on the computer, three hours later. One child in the carpool forgets his epi-pen so we turn around to get that. Child 2 forgets his lunch so mom has to rush back, cursing under her breath the whole time wondering why he can't just learn to eat frog's legs. Hell, it's a delicacy in some places. Child 3 gets off the computer to get a "snack" and leaves the kitchen looking like something out of an episode of "America's Test Kitchen Hoarders." And that's just the morning.

Pickup in the afternoon is even more of a cluster with the added benefit of sweaty, smelly kids in the car. And even though they were together all day, they must yell at each other, recounting the day's activities and events at the highest decibel level possible. Then, of course, they all start making plans about which house they are going to for the rest of the day. Or the pool, which entails wet bathing suits and pool towels inevitably ending up on the bedroom floors. Whichever house they end up at (hopefully not the America's Test Kitchen Hoarder's house), they are all ravenous and go through every industrial sized box of crap that was just purchased on a $350 Costco run.

We live in a neighborhood with a park and a pool. Why can't kids simply entertain themselves with these things? Or the basketball hoop in our driveway? I'm all for some structured activities but I think today we have gone way overboard. Not to mention the cost. It seems like come April, all I do is open up my checkbook and write another camp deposit check.

Summer also brings with it an endless stream of happy hours and outdoor drinking time. From adult sippy cups at the pool to evenings sitting around the fire, pit drinking. Not an easy time for a recovering alcoholic. Just as you have survived and put the tough holiday season behind you, here comes summer with all its temptation. And whether the kids go to camp and you are crazed with the logistics, or they stay home and drive you batty, you're pretty much ready for a drink at the end of the day. So I'm off to invent some fun summer mocktails that I can spend this last bit of spring perfecting. Maybe that's an idea for a new camp for junior: Kids' Mocktail Bartender Camp.

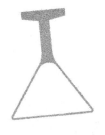

POOR ME SOME WHINE

I went into downtown Washington, D.C. today to have lunch with three women I worked with nearly 25 years ago. I still can't get it through my head that I can say I did anything as far back 25 years ago. (Yes, I worked when I was five years old). I hadn't seen them since I "came out" about my alcoholism. I know they read my blog so they are aware of my sobriety.

We met at an old favorite Mexican restaurant and I watched the waiters bringing margaritas, cold beers and shots of tequila to other diners. The cold beers looked really good. So did the margaritas. The tequila shots seemed a bit much even for me, an alcoholic, on a normal Wednesday afternoon. I thought about how in the old days, pre-sobriety, I would have been knocking back margaritas without giving it a second thought. But my friends all ordered non-alcoholic drinks, as did I.

I used to drive into DC from Northern Virginia every day when I worked as a lobbyist. Today, I felt like I was driving to Mars. Driving in the city brought a tsunami of memories as I passed bars I frequented, restaurants where I wined and dined colleagues and offices I visited for meetings, usually hungover. The liquor store near my old office was still there. Always a convenient place to pick up bottles of wine for Christmas gifts for others, or bottles of something stronger for Hangover Thursday gifts for myself.

The memories were both good and bad. Certainly many laughs and lots of good times. But also lots of mistakes and escapades I'd rather forget. The flood of memories came just after a string of several big disappointments the past two days. Suffice it to say that I had gotten my hopes up for a few things only to be slammed back down. In addition, a friend relapsed. And I have a nasty sinus infection. And none of my summer clothes fit. So my point with all this whining is what, you ask?

Any of these things on their own would be enough to feel like a kick in the stomach, but the perfect storm of crap that has blown in the last few days has me thinking how nice a big (huge) drink would be right now. It's that swirling around of so many different feelings in my head (much like the swirly margaritas I drooled over today at lunch) that makes it tough as an alcoholic. I used to drink to get all these feelings in check, or, more accurately, to get them to go the fuck away. I drank to numb, so I didn't have to actually feel the feelings. But now I do.

While feeling the bad feelings hurts (immensely sometimes), feeling the good ones can be an inexplicable joy. Memories fall into the same category. And the farther along I get in my recovery, the more memory bubbles that keep popping up. As much as my head hurts at times like this, and I'm not sure what to do with all these feelings since I no longer wash them down with booze, I'd still rather feel the ups and downs than not feel anything.

Yes, I know that life is full of disappointments. And yes, I understand that I just need to suck it up and put on my big girl panties. But sometimes I need to whine. And whining is better than wining. So thanks for letting me.

"Maturity is a bitter disappointment for which no remedy exists, unless laughter could be said to remedy anything."
— **Kurt Vonnegut**

ATTITUDE OF GRATITUDE

This is a very bittersweet weekend for me. Memorial Day weekend was the last time I drank, three years ago, on a girls' trip to NYC. It's the kickoff to summer, and right now the sun is shining brightly and it's beautiful outside. Last night as I drove kids to various activities, I couldn't help but notice all the people in our neighborhood who were sitting outside, enjoying the evening with a nice cold beverage. Visiting with neighbors, coming out after a long, cold winter. There are certainly going to be challenges for me this weekend. But I'm so much stronger now than this same weekend one year into my sobriety, even two.

For some reason, anniversaries of sobriety are hard for me. I get very anxious and squirmy. I've written about that on my one-year and two-year celebrations of my recovery. There's great potential for "stinkin thinkin," as they say. Potential for me to think that I've made it this far and that now I would be okay "just having one drink." Or potential to say that I've made it this long, that's enough. Vivid memories of all the fun I had in NYC that weekend come rushing back. But so do the haunting visions of my hands shaking at lunch until I got a glass (or six) of wine in me and nearly throwing up on stage at a Broadway show (a story for another day).

And I'll never forget sitting on the street corner in New York, at four in the morning, finally admitting to my friend that I was an alcoholic. That same friend hasn't missed a single day, now three years later, with the same text every morning checking on me. That's pretty high up there on my gratitude list.

Other friends have continued to hold me up, support me and carry me when times got tough and the power of this cunning, baffling disease tried to overtake me. They wouldn't let it. I'm grateful to them and especially to my sponsor, who is even able to simply sense when I am having a difficult time and shows up at my doorstep. And it goes without saying (obviously not if I'm saying it) that I couldn't do this without the love and support of my family. To have my thirteen-year old daughter tell me that she's proud of me means the world to me. Can you say "gratitude?"

Thanks for the comments on my blog pieces, the pats on the back and the kind words. And special thanks to the friend who pulled up yesterday while I was walking my youngest home from school and handed me a big, beautiful bouquet of flowers from her garden and a lovely handwritten note (yes, people actually still do that) of congratulations and encouragement. It meant a great deal to me and I'm very grateful for caring friends.

So I won't lock myself away in my bedroom this weekend, pulling the covers over my head to avoid all the temptations. I'll celebrate my son's birthday today—present, clear-headed, not hungover, and at peace. And I'll remember it when I wake up tomorrow morning too.

Most of all, let's not forget what this weekend is all about. A heartfelt thank you to those who have served our county and humbled remembrance of those who gave their lives. Freedom is way up there on my gratitude list too. Happy Memorial Day.

"As we express our gratitude, we must never forget that the highest appreciation is not to utter words, but to live by them."
— **John F. Kennedy**

MISUNDERSTANDING BEING MISUNDERSTOOD
PART I

There used to be a time when the weekends brought about a deep exhale and a break from the chaos of the week. The exhale used to come with imbibing large quantities of alcohol. For most people, weekends kicked off on Friday afternoon/evening. For me, I was usually well lit by then. Weekends are now chock-full of sports and kid activities. This particular week AND weekend were rough.

I went to my youngest son's end-of-season soccer party the other night. It was held at the coach's house and I didn't know most of the other parents of the kids on the team. I was already having a tough day when I walked out to the patio and saw everyone drinking cold Coronas with limes. Ugh. I was so tempted to do a 180 and high tail it out of there. But I didn't. I decided I needed to suck it up for my kid's sake and stay.

The hostess offered me some sparkling water, knowing I don't drink, and I gladly accepted. Having something in my hand immediately upon getting to a party is usually helpful. She saw me fidgeting and could tell how uncomfortable I was and said she would understand if I needed to go. Isn't this supposed to be easier now that I have three years of sobriety under my belt?? I guess the fact that I could sit down surrounded by people I didn't know, with no liquid courage in me to get to know them, while they were drinking cold beers, shows that I have come a long way. There's no way I would have been able to endure that situation a year ago.

I started talking to the couple sitting next to me and we went through the usual round of DC-area pleasantries—where you were from, what you did for work, where you went to school, etc. I shared that I used to be a lobbyist and they asked if I would ever want to go back. I told them no, because I didn't want to put myself back into a career that involved social functions morning, noon and night. I added that I was considering going back to work, I just wasn't sure doing what. Then I went on further and opened myself up for the conversation that ensued. I told them that I am currently a writer, that I have a blog and that I am hopefully publishing a book. On what they asked. A perfectly reasonable question, and one for which I'm going to have to work on having a better answer. I stumbled a little bit, but managed to convey to them that my blog was about my personal journey into recovery and sobriety. That I want to raise awareness about alcoholism among women just like me and that it's a huge problem in our society that is rarely talked about.

I waited nervously to see what their response was going to be. They seemed quite interested and followed up with numerous questions. While I felt like I was in the hot seat, I was well aware of the fact that I put myself there. If I'm going to wear my *Sobrietease* hat out in public, talk about my blog, and wear a necklace with a recovery symbol, I have to be able to be held accountable and not babble like an idiot or be at a loss for words when asked about these things. In fact, a woman at a golf tournament recently asked me about my necklace. You would have thought I was speaking Swahili back to her. I literally made no sense and told her that I forgot what the symbol stood for. Well done, jackass.

Others around us at the party were half-listening but I could tell that when they realized what the subject matter was, they didn't want to join in the conversation. The couple wished me well with my writing and said they would check out my blog. I hope they have.

On Saturday night, my husband and I went to a 50th birthday party for a very dear friend. It was a lovely party and I had been looking forward to it. As soon as we walked in, however, that social anxiety I used to keep at bay with my liquid courage grabbed a hold of me and nearly choked me. Once again, I quickly got some sparkling water from the bar to have something in my hand. Everyone was drinking. The smell of red wine wafted through the air and right into my nose, almost poking at me with every inhale. I tried to talk to a few people but was very uncomfortable. I didn't know if I would be able to stay long but wanted to be there to celebrate with my friend. When I started to feel some "stinking thinking" coming on, I immediately texted my sponsor. She asked if I could get out of there if I was struggling. I told her I could, but I was trying to be a big girl and stay. She told me to keep her posted and I went back to the party.

I saw a familiar face—a mother of one of the girls on my daughter's lacrosse team and felt a huge sigh of relief. She knows I don't drink and I would be comfortable talking to her for a bit. Someone else I was talking to wasn't drinking either, trying to stay in good shape for an early morning commitment. And here's where the misunderstanding that so many people have about alcoholism steps in. People who aren't drinking for the night, for whatever reason—they may be the designated driver or have to be up early (and not hungover) for something—try to rationalize why I can or cannot drink. There's the camp of people who say "I'm not drinking tonight and I don't see what the big deal is. This isn't so hard. Why is it so hard for you not to drink?" Then there's the other camp: "It's been three years. I don't understand why you can't just control it and have one or two drinks then stop." How I wish that any of that were true. Well, actually, some of it is true. I'm sure it isn't so hard for you not to drink on a given night. But for me, it is. It's actually very hard when every which way I turn I see and smell alcohol and watch it being consumed happily.

As for the questions of why can't I just have one or two drinks then stop, if I had the answer to that, I'd be beyond rich. The millions of alcoholics who ask that same question wish they had the answer to that as well. We are alcoholics. We cannot just "have one or two drinks." Maybe some days, we can. But on most days, one or two leads to nine or ten. Once we put alcohol into our systems, the disease is triggered. The switch is turned on, and as I have said before, my "off" switch is broken. Alcoholism has been described as both an obsession of the mind and a physical addiction. That first sip feeds the physical addiction and the obsession of the mind immediately follows. Alcoholics are powerless over alcohol.

When I am at a party, I miss what alcohol used to do for me. Caroline Knapp describes it perfectly in her book *Drinking: A Love Story*:

> *"That may be one of liquor's most profound and universal appeals to the alcoholic: The way it generates a sense of connection to others, the way it numbs social anxiety and dilutes feelings of isolation, gives you a sense of access to the world. You're trapped in your own skin and thoughts; you drink; you are released, just like that One drink, and the bridge—so elusive in the cold, nerve-jangled sensitivity of sobriety—appears, waiting only to be crossed."*

Trapped in my own skin. That is a perfect description. The stigma of alcoholism isn't going away any time soon. Many people don't see it as a disease but rather a weakness of character—that I can't stop because I have no self-restraint or limited self-control. I wish I could explain it as eloquently as Knapp does:

> *"Alcoholism seemed more to me like a moral issue than a physical one. This is one of our culture's most basic assumptions about the disease and one of its most destructive: we figure that drinking too much is a sign of*

weakness and lack of self-restraint; that it's bad; that it can be overcome by will."

For those who ask me if I will ever go back to drinking, and I know people who have, even after 18 years of sobriety, I will once again quote Knapp:

"Science may also explain why relapse rates are so high: those neurological reward circuits have extremely long and powerful memories, and once the simple message— alcohol equals pleasure—gets imprinted into the drinker's brain, it may stay there indefinitely, perhaps even a lifetime. Environmental cues, the sight of a wineglass, the smell of gin, a walk past a favorite bar—can trigger the wish to drink in a heartbeat, and they often do.

"Once you've crossed the line into alcoholism, the percentages are not in your favor: there appears to be no safe way to drink again, no way to return to a normal, social, controlled drinker."

Hopefully that helps address some of the misunderstanding. I don't blame people for not getting it. Why should you be expected to know these things if you aren't an alcoholic? I hope that part of what I can do with this book is help put aside some of the misconceived notions and educate people who want to understand this disease better. I'd love to hear from you—what questions do you have about alcoholism? What would you like to ask an alcoholic? I can address them in my next blog piece or future book. I don't have all the answers by any stretch of the imagination but I can share my own experiences.

"Misunderstanding must be nakedly exposed before true understanding can begin to flourish."
- **Philip Yancey**, *The Bible Jesus Read*

MISUNDERSTANDING BEING MISUNDERSTOOD
PART II

The most basic question I receive from my blog posts is how did I know I had a problem? The simple answer is that I knew that I was powerless over alcohol and that my life had become unmanageable. Conveniently, this is Step 1. Drinking had gone from enjoyment to need. Band Aid to crutch. Occasionally to almost-daily. White (wine) to black(outs). I drank to celebrate every occasion and to give myself liquid courage when I needed it. I drank when I was sad so I could wallow further in my depression. I drank when I was angry to try to make the anger go away. I drank when I was happy to take it to a higher level of joy. I drank when I was anxious, scared, lonely, proud, embarrassed... you get the idea. Once I started, the concept of moderation flew out the window. My "off" switch was broken. I drank before I went out to an event, on my way there, and when I got home. I thought I would just have a glass of wine while I made dinner and it inevitably turned into a bottle or more. I knew it had taken over my life.

Another good question: how and when did I know I needed to stop drinking? I've shared before how ashamed I was when my daughter asked me why I didn't remember something we talked about on a particular evening. And I remember how badly I felt when I was in bed, too hungover to do normal things with my kids. Then there was watching my hands shake until I got some wine in me at lunch in NYC. I think all of these things bubbled up inside and culminated in me coming clean to a friend who lost her husband to alcoholism. Even after I got sober, there were days when I had terrible cravings and told her I wanted a drink and she responded, "Go ahead, have a drink. The last time I touched my husband's hand it was cold." I don't mean to be totally morbid here, but this disease is no joke. I need my kids and the people I care about to know and understand that alcohol kills. It destroys your body and carves out a path of destruction throughout your entire life.

More than one person has asked what they should do if they know someone who they think may be an alcoholic or have a drinking problem. I hate to be the bearer of bad news, but no matter how much you want to help someone, you can't until they want it and are willing to help themselves. Getting sober is something no one can do for us, but also something that we cannot do alone. I have friends who knew I had a drinking problem long before I admitted it and either said they felt guilty about not doing anything to help or said that they knew if they tried to talk to me about it, our relationship would change and I might just try to hide my drinking from them. Until I was ready, no one could have done anything. Can you sit down with a family member or friend and tell them you are concerned? Absolutely. And that may be just what they need to push them to go get help.

Several people wanted to know if they are having a party, happy hour or event where there will be alcohol, is it better not to say anything to me because it would probably be hard for me to be there or if they should invite me anyway. Great question and I could see how people may not know what to do when they are trying to be sensitive. For me, I would definitely prefer to be invited and be given the chance to make the choice myself whether I attend or not. I have good days and bad days, just like everyone else, but on a bad day, being around alcohol may just be too tempting. On good days, I'm happy to go and be with friends. I may not be able to stay too long however, so please don't take that personally.

Another thing that shouldn't be taken personally is if I attend some events and not others. Again, it depends on how I'm feeling that particular day/night. And, what's really important to understand here is that alcoholics are supposed to avoid triggers—people, places and things that remind them of their drinking. It may not be too hard to handle one of those, but a perfect storm with a combo of all three can be both overwhelming and dangerous.

What do I do when I get a really bad craving and think that I just can't do it any more? Well, other than think of my friend telling me about her husband's cold hand, I adhere to some other good advice that was given to me: think the drink through. Think it all the way through. Not just how good that drink may taste, but what happens after that first sip? After that first drink? There would be many more. And how would I feel about throwing away three years of sobriety? How guilty would I feel? Would I be able to look my kids in the face? All these things help me when I think about picking up a drink.

I have to remember that while I am learning all this as I go, my family and many of my friends are as well. If it's your first time dealing with someone who has a problem with addiction, you may have lots of questions. Very early on in my sobriety, I wrote a piece called "How To..." about how to be friends with an alcoholic. Interestingly enough, on this journey, I'm learning how to be a good friend to this alcoholic as well.

"He who asks a question is a fool for five minutes; he who does not ask a question remains a fool forever."
– Chinese proverb

YOU SAY IT'S YOUR BIRTHDAY

Some people say that their birthdays are really no big deal to them. Not me. I think that my birthday should be a national holiday. Ticker-tape parade, fireworks, the whole nine yards. I like to try to drag my birthday out into at least a week-long celebration. The other day that ranks way up there, and is like a second birthday to me, is my sobriety date. In fact, many in recovery consider that date to be their birth day—the day they came into their new life. So that you have enough time to plan, my sobriety date is May 28, 2012.

My birthday was two days ago and I had a wonderful day. And it's shaping up to be a fantastic extended celebration. My husband surprised me with an overnight stay-cation at our favorite local hotel. My daughter cooked up an amazing dinner for me, and a few close friends, including my sponsor, joined us to celebrate. Other friends I will get to see for lunch or coffee this week for my prolonged birthday pageant. So thank you for all the well wishes, the flowers, emails, texts and Facebook posts. Very much appreciated. I hope any bank or store closings weren't too much of an inconvenience for anyone.

We also went to a lovely party this past weekend to celebrate a friend's 40th birthday. In the past three years, I have pretty much avoided events like this, knowing that I would be surrounded by lots of drinking. I wanted to put on my big girl panties and go to this one. The act didn't go unnoticed, as the birthday girl told me that it meant a great deal to her that I went. Made me feel good about my decision. When I walked in, I was pretty nervous and was anxiously wringing my hands and fidgeting.

My husband went to the bar to get me a mocktail so that I would have something to drink in my hands immediately. While he was at the bar, the husband of one of my dear friends kept me company and helped calm my nerves. It was nice to actually be out and be social for a change. I've kept to myself and hunkered down with my family so much during my recovery, it was good to branch out a little.

Things got a little tough for me when the restaurant staff started passing out champagne for the toast, but I moved away from the tray of flutes and my friend went to get me a glass of water to toast with. The evening culminated with an amazing fireworks display celebrating the city of Alexandria's birthday. I know that they were really for my birthday though.

No one gets to choose their birth date, but we can certainly choose our sobriety date. It's the day when we vow to stop drinking. The day we decide to turn our life around. The day we wave the white flag and sometimes fall to our knees begging for help. Each day sober after that date is a miracle and something to be celebrated. That's why I count my days. 1,144 to be exact. 1,144 days without a drop of alcohol. Some days are easy, and some days are brutally difficult. In a way, every one of those days is like a birthday for me. It's a day that I gain strength from my sobriety and grow in a way I wouldn't if I continued to be stifled by my drinking.

Only 316 more days to go until I hit 4 years and get that shiny coin. When I struggle and doubt myself and fear I can't make it, I'll try to remember the new person I gave birth to that day in NYC when gave up alcohol for good and finally ripped off the bandage. And those 316 days can only be done one way: one day at a time.

SET FREE

"If you love something, set it free.
If it comes back, it is yours.
If it doesn't, it never was."
– Unknown

There is some confusion over the authorship of the quote above. Many attribute it to Richard Bach, a novelist born in 1936, while others say it is from an unknown source. Regardless, its meaning is broad and deep. It's particularly applicable to my life right now. Someone lovingly "cut me loose" to stand on my own two feet and gain the strength I need to stay sober. It hurt at the time, and left me quite bewildered, but now that I look back, I can see it clearly and understand why.

No matter what our issues are in life, we all deal with some amount of codependency. Melody Beattie, author of several books on the topic says, "There are almost as many definitions of codependency as there are experiences that represent it." One simple definition is excessive emotional or psychological reliance in a relationship. There's an expression I hear often in the rooms that says, "detach with love." That's a healthy, admirable way to deal with codependency, though often much easier said than done.

While I have had a great deal of support throughout my recovery, I leaned quite heavily on one particular person who had a personal history with the other side of alcoholism. She got the texts when I longed for a drink. I turned to her to keep me from jumping off that ledge back into the world of alcohol. She had to listen to me whine and ask why I couldn't have a drink. And I realize now that that's an awful lot to put on any one person.

In another miraculous example of how God works, my decision to grow up and stop leaning so heavily on this person seemed to coincide almost exactly with when she decided it was time to cut me loose. She knew that I needed to develop the right tools to stay sober. More importantly, she understood that the only person who could keep me sober was me. And I knew that it was unfair to continue to lean so heavily on her, especially as she had her own trials and tribulations to deal with.

So what happened when she "detached with love?" I got my wings. I learned to stand on my own two feet and use the helpful instruments that I've acquired in my sobriety. I turned to my awesome sponsor and attended more meetings. I picked up some recovery literature. I learned to pray and to ask for help, and to turn things over to my *HP* (Higher Power).

Our friendship is stronger and deeper now and no longer allows alcoholism to dominate it. So to my friend, thank you for caring enough to let me find my own strength and plant my feet firmly underneath me. HP has now given me the strength and tools to help others. And to all the people I lean on heavily, thank you for being there for me throughout this journey.

"Taking care of myself is a big job.
No wonder I avoided it for so long."
– **Anonymous**

LESSONS FROM THE PAST

Sometimes I catch myself getting just a little too cocky with my sobriety and slipping into a false sense of security. The great thing about writing my blog is that I can use it to smack some sense back and scare the crap out of myself. In doing so, hopefully I can help a few others out there do the same. When we get complacent, don't get to as many meetings as we should (for whatever reason) and think that we're in a good place and feeling strong in our sobriety, it's an excellent time to look at the way we used to be and how we never want to be again.

As I wrote in one of my earlier pieces, "Misunderstanding Being Misunderstood," I shared that many people asked me how and when I knew I had a problem with alcohol. I can only share what the signs were for me, yours may be much different.

I thought I was just a social drinker who, on occasion, drank a little too much. Ok, a lot too much. But when I look back and see things clearly now, I can see how things turned and how the disease progressed. I used to think how nice a drink was going to taste when 5pm rolled around. The anticipation of that drink started taking over a greater part of my consciousness. That anticipation turned into a longing. That longing turned into a need. That "occasional social drink" turned into a must-have, even if I was by myself.

I used to look forward to pouring that first glass of wine while I made dinner for our family. Sometimes I would sip it slowly, return the bottle to the refrigerator and continue to cook and listen to my music. As my alcoholism progressed, that glass turned into the bottle, which I would bury among the empties in the recycling bin so my husband wouldn't know I had already consumed an entire bottle by myself before he came home from work. When friends stopped by, it seemed as if I had a free pass and it was okay that we polished off a whole bottle—even if I had three or four glasses of it and my friend had only one.

Some days when I wasn't quite ready to go to wine yet, I would make a stronger drink first. A Cosmo, gin or vodka and tonic, whatever, to prime the pump. Then I would go to the "lighter stuff" like wine or occasionally beer. Regardless, by the time we sat down to dinner I usually had quite a decent buzz going. But with that decent buzz came a not so decent version of me. I had a very short fuse and a very bad temper. The littlest things would set me off. I was not kind to my husband or my kids, and I focused all my attention on myself and where and when my next drink was going to come from.

I would, of course, have to continue to drink while I cleaned up the kitchen after dinner. Sometimes I thought it was a great idea to pick up the phone and call someone since I had the booze babble going. That or email people. That was brilliant as well. At least when you ramble on to someone on the phone the words are out and gone. Writing them down allows your drunken dribble to endure and get sent back to you for deciphering. And embarrassment.

After the calls and emails, it was bedtime or, more accurately, time to pass out. No telling my kids stories or tucking them in because I was too wasted and too self-centered. Sometimes I even passed out in my clothes. The days when I used to wear contact lenses were especially lovely, since I would wake up with them glued to my eyeballs. No conversations with my husband, unless it was an incoherent ranting about something. No watching a show or movie together. He was busy doing the tucking in and story-telling.

The next morning would inevitably start with a miserable hangover and those first few minutes upon waking were spent trying to piece together the night before. I needed to figure out how bad the hangover was, try to recall how much I drank and who I called or emailed. I would have too bad of a headache and upset stomach to eat any kind of normal breakfast, and I barked at my kids while doing the minimal amount of work necessary to feed them and get them dressed and ready for school. On really bad mornings, I would simply go back to bed and nurse my hangover all day. On days when I had to actually function, I threw some very cold water on my face, grabbed my Diet Coke and struggled to get through what I had to. I've got to believe that people could smell booze coming out of my pores and breath. But it was always just laughed off as yet another hangover.

And the cycle went on, waiting until 5pm to crack open that next bottle. If a friend stopped by earlier, after school, it was a good excuse to start my drinking day even sooner. How did I feel throughout this whole period? Like absolute crap. Physically and emotionally. I was depressed and drank alcohol, a depressant, which I told myself actually helped me to feel better. I was miserable and I was making everyone around me miserable too. A few friends tried to tell me that I had to get a grip on my drinking but I brushed them off completely, telling myself that they had no idea what they were talking about. I remember looking in the mirror, morning and night, and not liking what I saw at all.

Fast forward to today, 1,172 days since I've had a drink, and I can honestly tell you that I feel a thousand times better. Well maybe 1,172 times better. I feel better all around. I am here for my kids and my husband. And my friends. I start each day fresh, usually on my knees thanking my HP for another day sober and healthy. I end each day being able to look in the mirror and be proud of who I see looking back at me. I remember what I say and email to friends and family.

And I need to remind myself, as I'm doing here, that my sobriety is a daily reprieve, and can be gone in one split second if I take a sip of a drink. It's a little more difficult to be cocky when I remind myself of the times I spent doubled over and throwing up. My daughter asked me once when she was really sick with a stomach virus if that's how I felt when I would be sick from drinking too much. I told her yes, only much worse. She said she couldn't understand how I could ever intentionally make myself that ill. I can't either. But thankfully, those days are gone.

"We are made wise not by the recollection of our past,
but by the responsibility for our future."
– George Bernard Shaw

MOCKTAIL MANIA, PART I

When Friday night rolls around and my friends are all picking up their first cocktails of the weekend, I'm usually fixing myself a seltzer with lime or, if I'm really feeling crazy, mixing it with some cranberry juice. Three years and almost three months into my sobriety, that's getting old.

Many of you will remember that in February, to celebrate my 1,000th day of sobriety, we hosted a mocktail party. We held a contest to see who could come up with the best mocktail name and the best tasting mocktail. There were some very clever entries. (See "One Thousand Shades of Sober," page 101).

I'm happy to report that some very clever people have taken the concept a step farther and started a company called *Mocktails*. They currently have four different flavors of nonalcoholic beverages on the market: *Karma Sucra* (Cosmopolitan), *Sevilla Red* (Sangria), *The Vida Loca* (Margarita) and *Scottish Lemonade* (Whiskey Sour). I had the pleasure of sampling two of them this weekend.

They come in their own glass shakers, ready to go. All you have to do is add ice, shake and pour into your favorite glass. I will say that I had to pour a little out into a separate glass to fit the ice in—I'm not complaining though. I'd rather do that and have them fill the shaker up as much as possible than cut back on the amount. I invited two friends, also nondrinkers, over to do the taste tests with me.

There are many who participate in 12-step or other programs for recovery who are adamantly opposed to the concept of nonalcoholic beers or pseudo-cocktails. In fact, my therapist refers to them as "mental masturbation." I guess they feel that you are perpetuating the whole ritual and habit of drinking alcohol by drinking even a non-alcoholic beer (which does have a very small amount of alcohol in it). It still smells like a beer and looks like a beer. And pouring these Mocktails into martini glasses, they look like, well, cocktails. BUT, I did check with my sponsor and got the okay. We agreed that since there is NO alcohol in the new Mocktails and since we are often looking for something new and creative to drink while others enjoy happy hour, we could give it a try.

We tried the *Sevilla Red* Sangria first. I poured some out into a separate glass, filled the shaker with some ice, put the top back on and shook away. It has been a long time since I shook a martini shaker. The sound did drum up some old memories for a split second. I unscrewed the top and poured some through the strainer into three very pretty martini glasses. Hey, I know that sangria isn't supposed to be served in martini glasses but give me a break somewhere.

I think it is fair to say that all three of us expected a sickeningly sweet concoction that was going to leave our lips puckered. We were all very pleasantly surprised. After the first few sips, we decided to add some cut up fruit into the glasses like true sangria. Even better. The shaker says it serves four, but we got almost 2 full glasses for all three of us.

Next, we moved on to *Karma Sucra*, their version of a virgin Cosmopolitan. Also sweet tasting without being overly sugary, but this one had a little bit of a medicinal taste to it. We added a little seltzer (watermelon and lime flavored) which gave it a smoother taste. These drinks are only 50 calories per serving, with no artificial flavors or colors, no preservatives, no high fructose corn syrup, gluten free, BPA free, allergen free, and Kosher! And, for those of you who don't have a broken "off" switch like me, feel free to add alcohol to them if you want.

Bottom line: I'm very happy to have an alternative to seltzer now to drink at happy hour. Having the drinks did not make me want alcohol at all. I was happy to have the yummy taste and the pretty drink without it. And happy to wake up without a hang-over the next day. Bravo to the Mocktails folks!

LIFE OUTSIDE THE COMFORT ZONE

I have a magnet on my refrigerator that says, "Life begins outside the comfort zone." A very dear friend suggests doing one thing every day out of your comfort zone. I started to think about my journey through recovery and thought about how much of it has been outside what I would consider my comfort zone.

From the very moment when we admit our weaknesses, in my case being powerless over alcohol, we become vulnerable and take a giant leap of faith outside our comfort zone. Alcohol was my comfort zone. I turned to it when I was sad and depressed, I turned to it when I was happy and wanted to celebrate, I turned to it for pretty much everything. Admitting that my life had become unmanageable because of alcohol was step one out of that territory.

The next monumental step for me was walking into the rooms of AA. I'll never forget how desperate I was for help (often called the "gift of desperation") but how scared I was to walk into my first meeting. I sat outside in my car on the phone with my friend who told me to go in because I would be with people who understood exactly what I was going through. She was right. Next step out of my comfort zone was saying the words out loud, "My name is Martha and I am an alcoholic." I could barely get them out of my mouth.

As I continued on my path to recovery, there were several other turns away from what had become my norm. Asking someone to be my sponsor. Sharing at a meeting. Leading a meeting. Working the twelve steps. Surrendering and turning things over to my Higher Power. Asking for the "serenity to accept the things I cannot change, the courage to change the things I can, and the wisdom to know the difference." Making a searching and fearless moral inventory of my character defects. Making a list of all the people I had harmed when I was drinking. Making amends to those people. And now, trying to help others as they go through this process or similar ones. It doesn't have to be alcohol. Whatever your demons are, having the guts to face them and working to overcome them inevitably takes you out of your comfort zone.

As human beings, familiarity and routine are comforting to us. Breaking out of those can be scary, sometimes terrifying. But without making a decision as to which path to take at the crossroads, and often choosing the more difficult one, we cannot grow. Another friend of mine often says, "Sometimes the only form of transportation available to us is a giant leap of faith." We can stay on the path of what is familiar and comfortable, even though in my case it could be fatal, or we can take that road filled with potholes and bumps which leads to a better life.

Growth and emotional maturity are the rewards of that step outside the comfort zone. But it takes work. Michael Barbarulo said, "God has given you the power and desire to change but you still need to be willing to do the work. Doing the work means facing your fears and getting out of your comfort zone." It has also been said that courage is not a lack of fear, but rather a mastery of fear with the help of your Higher Power. Although the work can be challenging to say the least, we don't have to do it alone. We can use the resources available to us to smooth the potholes and bumps in the road and help us along our journey.

LIQUID COURAGE DOWN THE DRAIN

I had to speak at an event for work this past weekend in front of 100 people. Normally, I would have pounded a drink (or several) beforehand to calm my nerves—a little liquid courage if you will. Now, almost 3½ years into my sobriety, I had to do this without my usual crutch. Was I nervous? Yes. Very. But somehow when I got up to the podium, I managed to stay calm and actually speak coherently. It certainly helped to have so many friendly faces in the crowd—a sincere thank you to my friends who were able to make it. I truly appreciate the support.

I started a new job about 2 months ago. I'm working as the Executive Director of the National Breast Center Foundation. It was started by a local doctor a little over a year ago to ensure that low-income and uninsured women have access to screenings, mammograms and treatment for breast cancer. Turns out that the DC area, where I live, has the highest incidence and mortality rate from breast cancer in the country. It also has one of the highest rates of late stage breast cancer in the nation. It is truly a privilege to work for someone who is actually trying to make a difference and address this crisis.

It's been over ten years since I hung up my hat as a lobbyist for the telecommunications industry. I left when my middle child turned one to stay home and be a mom. Best decision I ever made. But there were definitely days when I missed the interaction with other adults and putting on real clothes to go somewhere other than my laundry room. I truly enjoyed my work but something had to give. I felt as though I was doing everything half-assed and nothing well. There are heated debates about both sides of the concept of being able to have it all as a woman—career and family—but that is a blog post for another day. Back to liquid courage.

My former job as a lobbyist involved a great deal of drinking and socializing. Lots of receptions, dinners, fundraisers, etc. And I drank through all of them. I downed my liquid courage before I had to walk into a social situation where I didn't know anyone. A drink at a business lunch helped facilitate the conversation, or so I thought. Drinks with colleagues after work were a common occurrence. Drinks on the golf course too. But now, 10 years since I worked and 3½ years sober, there is none of that. I'm on my own without the crutch of liquid courage.

I was very open and honest about my alcoholism when I applied for the job. It's pretty easy to find my blog and connect me to it. That's intentional. I explained when I interviewed that I am very forthcoming about being an alcoholic and about my blog. I do it so that others in similar situations will know they are not alone and to shed a little light on a subject that still isn't talked about enough in our society. One of the board members who interviewed me asked me flat out if I thought my alcoholism would affect my job. I said it would. It would make me better at it.

I know who I am and I am getting more comfortable in my own skin. I am finding my own voice and am able to use it without needing liquid courage to do so. Better to be open about being a recovering alcoholic than to have an employee who comes in trying to hide a miserable hangover. Or worse.

So here's to pouring that liquid courage down the drain. *Cheers.*

> *"I learned that courage was not the absence of fear but the triumph over it. The brave man is not he who does not feel afraid, but he who conquers that fear."*
> – **Nelson Mandela**

MOCKTAIL MANIA, PART II

We held another Mocktail Party this past weekend. Unlike the last party, where people created and named their own concoctions, drinks were provided this time by Mocktails Beverages, Inc., an awesome new company that makes delicious non-alcoholic beverages. Two of the company's cofounders, Ali and Jim, brought plenty of their product and served as bartenders for us for the evening. They were two of the nicest people you'd ever want to meet.

There are four flavors of Mocktails: *Scottish Lemonade* (like a Whiskey Sour), *La Vida Loca* (Margarita), *Karma Sucra* (Cosmopolitan) and *Sevilla Red* (Sangria). I did a review of them in a previous blog. The only one I hadn't tasted before was the *Scottish Lemonade*, and that turned out to be my favorite (and the favorite of many other people as well). The best thing about this product is that there are no artificial flavors, colors or preservatives, no high fructose corn syrup, they are gluten free, Kosher, all natural, allergen free, and BPA free. As I said in my earlier review, I expected them to be sickeningly sweet and they absolutely were not.

When I spoke to Mocktails President and Founder, Bill Gamelli, a few months ago, he told me why they started the company. He and a few college friends (including Jim) had members of their own families who found it difficult to find any good options when they were in social situations where most people were drinking alcohol. He said that the product is for those who want a different choice when they go out and aren't drinking alcohol. Take it from me, water and seltzer get a little boring. Whatever the reason someone isn't drinking alcohol—whether they are pregnant, an athlete in training, the designated driver that night, on medication that can't be mixed with alcohol, or, like me, an alcoholic—Mocktails can be a great choice. And for those who do want to drink, alcohol can be added to any of the four products.

When I first got sober, I pretty much hibernated in my house alone. I couldn't handle the idea of going somewhere and having to answer the questions of why I wasn't drinking. People were definitely used to my having a drink in my hand. What I finally know now is that no one really cares if I am drinking or not and it isn't a big deal to just say I'm not drinking. But back then I was scared and hanging on to my sobriety for dear life. If I had Mocktails back then, it would have been easier for me to socialize because people wouldn't have been able to tell if I was drinking or not and I wouldn't have had to deal with the questions.

Our party guests were all pleasantly surprised by the flavors of the Mocktails. We served them in the appropriate glass for each drink. Jim and Ali poured with smiles and explained to those who asked all about the product. It was a Saturday night and I was actually having a party at my house, not sitting in my pajamas reading a book as usual.

A huge thank you to Ali and Jim, as well as Bill and the rest of the team, and kudos on an excellent product. What they have created is so much more than just a non-alcoholic beverage— it's an open door to a whole new world of possibilities for the non-drinker.

"Creativity involves breaking out of established patterns in order to look at things in a different way."
– Edward de Bono

GIMME TWELVE STEPS

I used to love the Lynyrd Skynyrd song "Gimme Three Steps." I remember dancing to it with my friend Lisa in high school at her house while getting ready for a party. Inevitably, I drank too much and don't remember the rest of the night. The irony hit me when I realized today's dance for me would somehow revolve around a twelve step program, since that is such a huge focus of my life. In other words, you can gimme three steps, but I'll need nine more.

I've talked about the twelve steps to recovery before ("Slowly I Turned, Step by Step"). I feel like I'm treading on thin ice when I do because there are those diehards with respect to the anonymity aspect of AA who get extremely nervous when there is a mere mention of them. Like I am violating a secret code. As I have said before, I have the utmost respect for the program and wouldn't ever want to disrespect any of its rules. But it is easy to find the twelve steps anywhere on the Internet.

The wonderful thing about the twelve steps is that they can be applied to many problems in life, not just alcoholism. There are so many situations where I would be much better off if I would simply third-step them. The third step states that we "Made a decision to turn our will and our lives over to the care of God as we understood Him." Think about the Lord's prayer: "Thy will be done." THY will, not MY will. Turning things over to God (or whatever Higher Power you follow) brings about a whole new world of peace. Being able to recognize the things that are not in our control is not only humbling but pacifying. I've pretty much always been a worrier. Now I'm a warrior. I can't tell you the serenity that the third step has brought to my life.

Then there's the eleventh step: "Sought through prayer and meditation to improve our conscious contact with God, as we understood Him, praying only for knowledge of His will for us and the power to carry that out." If we are uncertain what God's will for us is, we can simply pray for that knowledge. And if we doubt our strength, we can simply pray for power. Look how much this simplifies life. Everyone should have some form of a twelve step program.

But perhaps the most helpful, and most difficult, is the fourth step: "Made a searching and fearless moral inventory of ourselves." Could you imagine a world where everyone did this, not just addicts or alcoholics? A searching and fearless moral inventory. A list of our good and bad. A real and honest look inside ourselves. If we can identify our own flaws and character defects, and then pray for God to remove these shortcomings (as we do in Step 7), we can become a better, new and improved person (Martha 2.0, as my friend calls me). But believe me, step four is not easy. For many, it opens up the closet to too many skeletons and demons that are just too difficult to deal with, especially sober. The good thing is, if you are able to get through step four, and then in step 5 admit them to yourself, to God and to another human being, you can leave the past behind you.

So that you don't have to go and search the internet, I'm going to list all *Twelve Steps of Alcoholics Anonymous* for your here. If you know someone in recovery, this will help you to understand what they are going through better. If you are just curious and wonder if these steps might be applicable to your life somehow, try them out.

The Twelve Steps

1. Admitted we were powerless over alcohol, that our lives had become unmanageable.

2. Came to believe that a power greater than ourselves could restore us to sanity.

3. Made a decision to turn our will and our lives over to the care of God as we understood Him.

4. Made a searching and fearless moral inventory of ourselves.

5. Admitted to God, to ourselves and to another human being the exact nature of our wrongs.

6. Were entirely ready to have God remove all these defects of character.

7. Humbly asked Him to remove our shortcomings.

8. Made a list of all persons we had harmed, and became willing to make amends to them all.

9. Made direct amends to such people wherever possible, except when to do so would injure them or others.

10. Continued to take personal inventory and when we were wrong promptly admitted it.

11. Sought through prayer and meditation to improve our conscious contact with God, as we understood Him, praying only for knowledge of His will for us and the power to carry that out.

12. Having had a spiritual awakening as the result of these Steps, we tried to carry this message to alcoholics, and to practice these principles in all our affairs.

Even step 12 advocates for practicing these principles in all our affairs. I try to carry this message to other alcoholics, as well as to other people who may benefit from it. Of course, you may not have any shortcomings or character defects, but I sure as hell do. But I'm working on them and I'm asking them to be removed.

I didn't give much attention to steps eight and nine—making a list of people we had harmed with our drinking and making amends to them. That's for another post. I wish I could just do a blanket apology here and say sorry to all those I hurt, but I can't. I need to do the work. But when it gets tough, I still may just ask you to gimme three steps towards the door.

"The journey of a thousand miles begins with a single step."
– Lao Tzu

BLACK(OUT) FRIDAY

The holidays can be a crazy time of year. For many, they bring up all kinds of memories—good and bad. For some, there is a struggle to search back into the recesses of our minds to see if we can even find the memories or if they are still as dark as the blackouts that may have enveloped them. For me, Thanksgiving reminds me of a few times I'd rather forget.

Thanksgiving was always a huge drinking day for me. I would start quite early with champagne or mimosas as family arrived and I cooked. I had a full glass of something for the rest of the day and night. Wine flowed throughout the Thanksgiving meal. Most people stopped drinking and had coffee with dessert, watched football, or took a walk or a nap, but I continued to drink. Didn't want to lose the buzz. We used to go to close friends for dessert where I welcomed the opportunity to have a plethora of new wines to "sample." But often by this point in the day or evening, I was slurring, stumbling or literally falling down drunk. How embarrassing to look back upon. What's even worse is to have to just imagine and wonder what I did when I passed that point and maybe even blacked out. I always laugh at meetings when people say they don't think they were blackout drinkers. How the hell would you know if you were—you certainly wouldn't remember?!

There were those totally inebriated Thanksgivings. One where I cried before I got up the courage to talk to my brother on the phone when he was in jail. One where I had a total meltdown in front of my friends about my unhappiness in my life and my marriage and said a bunch of things I still regret to my mom. Ones where I passed out in my wine-stained clothes, most likely leaving it to my husband to tell the kids that mommy is just really tired from all the cooking. Again, alcohol is a depressant. Adding that to an already depressed person is a recipe for disaster.

In just three more days, I'll have 3½ years of sobriety (God willing). One important thing that I have learned in that time is that I have a choice as to how I look back and how I move forward. Looking back, I can wallow in the miserable, drunken episodes, beat myself up and struggle to remember and relive the embarrassment. Or I can look back and use them to remind myself of a place I never want to return. Use them to "keep it green" as they say. And I can dig deep to remember the good times instead. The Thanksgivings where my grandparents were with us and inadvertently had us all cracking up. The Thanksgivings where we were all together. The Thanksgiving where my kids made little turkeys out of their hands and wrote the things that they were thankful for.

Going forward, instead of focusing all my attention on where my next drink is coming from, I can focus on the things for which I am truly grateful. That I'm not in that deep, dark depression but in a much better, happier, healthier place. That I am sober and present for my family. That I can wake up the day after Thanksgiving and not be completely hungover with a pounding headache or even still drunk. And that I am blessed with amazing friends who have been with me through thick and thin.

Happy Thanksgiving.

"Sometimes you will never know the true value of a moment until it becomes a memory."
– Dr. Seuss

RIGOROUS HONESTY

Here I am, 1308 days into my sobriety, and just plain pissed off. Pissed off that I still want to drink as badly as I do 3½ years later. Yes, the holidays are hard. And for many people, they are much more difficult than they are for me. People who have lost loved ones and desperately miss them during this season. People who find themselves all alone. People battling serious illnesses. But I am battling a serious illness. One that no one likes to talk about. Alcoholism is no joke. And frankly, it sucks.

There is drinking all around during the holiday season. I'm surrounded by it. I look at people enjoying their red wine and I salivate at the sight of it. When I'm feeling strong in my sobriety, working my program like I should, I am able to turn the other cheek and get on with whatever I'm doing. When I'm not where I should be in my sobriety, not going to enough meetings, not keeping in touch with my sponsor, that salivating turns into a desire, an urge to drink, that simply grows stronger. It almost takes on a life of its own.

When it does, I feel like it's an old friend that I miss very much. A friend that I have been forbidden from seeing again. I know deep down the bad things that will happen if I start hanging out with that friend again, yet I long for that camaraderie once more. Other people can drink, why can't I? I start to throw myself my own little pity party. It's not fair. Then the stinking thinking starts in. Maybe now, since I've been sober for a while, I'll be able to control my drinking. Never mind that it's pretty much never worked for anyone else, but somehow I think I'm different. I actually tried it before and went a while with my drinking "under control." It very quickly, however, spiraled out of control.

In the battle against alcoholism, it's literally all or nothing. There's a chapter in the *AA Big Book* entitled "How it Works" that says, "Half measures availed us nothing." To me, these are 5 of the most important words in the entire *Big Book*. You have to be all-in to successfully fight this disease. The chapter also says: "Rarely have we seen a person fail who has thoroughly followed our path. Those who do not recover are people who cannot or will not completely give themselves to this simple program, usually men and women who are constitutionally incapable of being honest with themselves. There are such unfortunates. They are not at fault; they seem to have been born that way. They are naturally incapable of grasping and developing a manner of living which demands rigorous honesty. Their chances are less than average."

Rigorous honesty. That's tough. Try it. You may even think that you are being completely honest with yourself but it's not as easy as it sounds. And even if you are completely honest with yourself, that's not enough. Steps 4 and 5 in AA are two of the toughest steps there are. Step Four states that we are to have: "Made a searching and fearless moral inventory of ourselves" and Step Five says we should have: "Admitted to God, to ourselves and to another human being the exact nature of our wrongs." Many people never make it past these steps. It's just too hard to deal with some of the skeletons in their closets. Some people think that just by being honest with themselves and identifying their character defects is enough. It's not. The program states that we must admit them to another human being. The *Big Book* says "if we skip this vital step, we may not overcome drinking. Time after time, newcomers have tried to keep to themselves certain facts about their lives... having persevered with the rest of the program, they wondered why they fell. We think the reason is they never completed their housecleaning. They took inventory all right, but they hung on to some of the worst items in stock. They only THOUGHT they had lost their egotism and fear; they only THOUGHT they had humbled themselves. But they had not learned enough of humility, fearlessness and honesty, in the sense we find it necessary, until they told someone else all their life story."

I've been stuck on Steps 4 and 5 for a while now. I thought that I had done Step 5 pretty thoroughly. But as I said, "pretty thoroughly" doesn't cut it. It's got to be done completely. I've shared some of "the exact nature of my wrongs" with my best friend, some with my sponsor and some with my therapist. But unfortunately, some still sit inside of me and until I deal with them, I may continue to be pissed off at how often I crave a drink. Rigorous honesty.

While the holidays are tough, the New Year brings with it new opportunities. I'm going to work on my fourth and fifth steps and continue on with the rest of the steps. I'm going to work my program thoroughly, completely, and honestly. I'm tired of the struggle with the cravings and tired of whining about trying to understand why I can't have a drink. I can't. I'm an alcoholic. And that's rigorous honesty right there.

"Can you honestly love a dishonest thing?"
– John Steinbeck

A BRIDGE OF SILVER WINGS

I hate New Year's Eve. I hated it when I was drinking and I hate it now that I'm sober. At least I could tolerate it more when I drank. But as an alcoholic, I considered it amateur night. What most people drank on New Year's Eve was about what I consumed on a normal day. And, as someone who suffers from depression, the end of the year wrap-ups and forced look back at my life always bring me down. The news channels faithfully play some sappy song and run through all of the people who have passed away throughout the year. People use New Year's Eve as an excuse to get stinking, obnoxiously drunk. You couldn't pay me enough money to stand squished between a zillion other people in NYC to watch a ball drop. What's the attraction? I don't know if there is an Ebenezer Scrooge equivalent for New Year's, but if so, I think I would fit the bill.

For the past few years, I've stayed home and just avoided the whole scene. It was too hard and too tempting that early in my sobriety. My friends invited me to their New Year's Eve parties, which I greatly appreciated, but I just couldn't do it. This year, I decided to go, at least for a little while. It was nice to be with friends in a beautiful house with delicious food and lots of warmth. But also lots of drinking. It got louder and louder. They were having a great time, drinking, dancing, eating, partying. Most of them told me that they were glad I came and that they understood that it must be hard for me to be around so much drinking. I left when I just knew I wasn't going to be able to be strong for that much longer, nowhere close to midnight.

I felt badly leaving, like a big party-pooper, and felt like I was cheating my family out of staying and having a good time. These are the times when it sucks to be an alcoholic. My son asked me this morning why we are always the first ones to leave the party. Ouch. But if I don't keep myself sober, I'd feel like I'm cheating my family out of a hell of a lot more.

Thank goodness this time of year, around the holidays, you can pretty much find a meeting any time, day or night. I knew it was important for me to go to a meeting yesterday, New Year's Eve, and I'm so glad I went. No matter how bad you think you've got it, there's always someone who is worse off. I heard several people talk about how rough 2015 was for them, and I mean rough. They were more than ready for the year to come to an end. Most importantly, I heard the speaker talking about how crucial it is to never forget the pain or the "gift of desperation" that brought us into the rooms of AA. I felt incredibly blessed to have somewhere to go where I could be with other alcoholics who get it. And I realized that my 2015 really wasn't so bad.

So I woke up this morning, a new day, a new year, ready for a fresh start. I can choose how I'm going to face this upcoming year and what my attitude will be. It's already off to a good start. I went to walk a friend's dogs and ran into a bunch of families playing kickball in the park. I joined them for a little while and had a great time. One of my friends there told me what she was feeding her family, a tradition of New Year's foods for "health and wealth" (black-eyed peas and collard greens). I told her I'd take all the health and wealth I could, and she showed up at my door a few hours later with a sample for us.

Hopefully now, the toughest parts of the holidays are behind me and I can stop my whining to you all. Thanks for being there to listen and for your encouragement to stay strong. I really appreciate it. For those of you out there who are still struggling, don't give up. It's much better on the other side of the bottle. Much better. Happy New Year.

"A bridge of silver wings stretches from the dead ashes of an unforgiving nightmare to the jeweled vision of a life started anew."

– Aberjhani, *Journey through the Power of the Rainbow: Quotations from a Life Made Out of Poetry*

I HAVE A DREAM…OR A FLAG

*"In the end we will remember not the words
of our enemies, but rather the silence of our friends."*
– Martin Luther King, Jr.

Most people remember Martin Luther King, Jr. for his "I Have a Dream" speech from August 28th, 1963. He had so many other memorable quotes, it's hard for me to choose just one for this piece. The one above really resonated with me. But on this weekend when we celebrate Reverend King, I am reminded of another remarkable civil rights figure, Rosa Parks. I had the distinct honor of meeting Ms. Parks back in 1991 at a Congressional Black Caucus event in Washington, D.C., which I attended with a very good friend of mine. Rosa Parks was nearly 80 years old and in a wheel chair, and I remember getting goose bumps when I got the chance to shake her small, frail hand.

Fast forward about fifteen years, when my daughter was in first grade. She told us one day that she was learning about Rosa Parks in school. I told her all about my encounter with Ms. Parks and what an honor it was for me to meet her, and encouraged her to share that story with her teacher and her classmates. I thought it would be pretty neat for a first grader to tell her class that her mom had met someone famous they were studying.

A few days went by, and I asked my daughter if she told her teacher and her classmates that I had met Rosa Parks. Her eyes welled up with tears and she said, "Yes, I did, but they didn't believe me." "What do you mean they didn't believe you? I met her! It was such a great privilege! I'll have to talk to your teacher." So the next time I was in her class volunteering, I broached the subject with her teacher.

Prepared to provide the details of my experience with Ms. Parks, I said to the teacher, "My daughter said she shared with you and the class that I met Rosa Parks and that you all didn't believe her. It's true. I did meet her. At Congressional Black Caucus in 1991. She was in a wheelchair..." I was prepared to go on but I realized I already sounded more than a little defensive. I shut up long enough for the teacher to speak and tell me this: "No, we didn't believe her. Because she told us you met Betsy Ross." Ouch. I may be old...but not THAT old.

"Each person must live their life as a model for others."
– Rosa Parks

IS IT TOO LATE NOW TO SAY SORRY?

Many people are familiar with the concept of alcoholics having to make amends. They may think it's as simple as going around and apologizing to those people you somehow screwed over or offended (or worse) in your prime drinking days. Not exactly. I thought about how nice it would be if I could just write a blanket apology in my blog for all the idiotic things I had done to various people and hope that they read it. I would venture to guess that my sponsor would veto that option.

Step 8 prepares us for our amends and says that we are to have "made a list of all persons we had harmed, and became willing to make amends to them all." Step 9 tells us to: "make direct amends to such people wherever possible, except when to do so would injure them or others." I'm not "officially" up to Steps 8 and 9 (as I've mentioned before, I've been stuck on Step 4 for quite some time. It's a really tough one: "Made a searching and fearless moral inventory of ourselves"). But I had a chance recently to make an amend that I knew I needed to make, so I seized the opportunity.

I have to admit that I was quite nervous, as I had no idea how it would be received. I'm incredibly fortunate that my first amends went very smoothly. It was to a dear friend from college. I'd prefer not to say what I did to screw things up, but let's just say it involved my behavior at his fraternity formal. Ugh. We had gone several years without speaking and I just attributed it to us both being busy and losing touch. It turned out that he was very upset with me. When I stopped drinking and saw things more clearly, I was able to look in the mirror and see the giant jackass that looked back at me.

I asked him to go to lunch. I wasn't sure how I was going to bring it up but HP works in wonderful ways—the opportunity was handed to me on a silver plate. I told him he looked great and he said he had cut way back on drinking and that had helped. It was like he rolled out the red carpet for my ninth step. I told him that I was now sober and that I was sincerely sorry for what I had done. Now was the tough part—waiting for the reaction. His eyes welled up with tears a little, he said how proud of me he was and that it was all "water under the bridge now." Exhale. Phew.

I don't expect them all to go that smoothly but hopefully many will. There are some that I can't make because the people are either gone or I have no idea where they are. There are some that can't be made because to do so would in fact "harm them or others." What can I do? Write a letter. Share it with my sponsor. Turn it over. And I will have to do those things to move forward in my sobriety. As it says in the "big book" of AA: "we will never get over drinking until we have done our utmost to straighten out our past."

So what should you do if you are on the other side of the amends—the one to whom the apology is made? First of all, please try to realize how hard it probably was for this person to come to you. You may be extremely pissed off with them because they left you stranded somewhere when they were drunk and forgot to meet you. You may be angry because they hit on your boyfriend when they were hammered. It might be much more serious than that—they may have ruined part of your life along with theirs. You may be furious for any number of reasons. Here's the thing: it's up to you what you do with that apology. You don't necessarily have to forgive them for them to move on and consider their job done. At least you know that they are trying to improve their lives, get sober and stay sober.

Ideally, you would try to make them comfortable through the difficult task. As I said, you may be very angry with them, but perhaps you are able to see them now and know that they were a different person then. A person who was under the spell of alcohol. A person with a progressive disease. How do you know if they are sincere? If they are truly working the steps, have a sponsor, going to meetings, and making an honest effort to not just stop drinking but to tackle the demons that led them to drink in the first place, give them a chance. If they have thoroughly done a fourth step, they are genuinely working toward making themselves better and healthier.

Is it too late now to say sorry? For me, in some instances, yes. But that doesn't mean I won't make amends where I can. And for this alcoholic, I consider a "living amends," making an effort every single day to be a better person, the most sincere way that I can show that I am truly sorry.

FINDING PEACE IN THE CHAOS

Life is a little chaotic and super busy, but all good. We held our Second Annual Mocktail Mania party a few weeks ago. Some really great and clever entries again this year. The winning drink, for both name and taste, was a take-off on a Moscow Mule: the Alexandria Ass. Delicious concoction and awesome name. I'm really happy that people get so into the mocktails and hope they know how much I appreciate the support.

This past weekend, I had what I consider a huge turning point in my sobriety. I had to attend a charity dinner with my boss. Not just a dinner, but a five-course meal with wine pairings. Perfect for an alcoholic. I tried turning my wine glass over, but the wait staff kept bringing new glasses with each pairing, already poured. I decided to offer the gentleman next to me my wines as they came. He asked me if I didn't like wine and I simply said that I did, just a little too much. After I slid a few glasses his way, he put his arm around me and said I was the best person he's ever sat next to at a wine dinner. The amazing thing was that being surrounded by all that wine didn't even bother me. In the earlier days of my sobriety, I would have been totally stressed out, sweating bullets and texting my sponsor for help. It's a huge relief to know how far I've come. I don't expect that it will always be that easy, or that I won't have cravings still, but I'll take this as a giant step forward.

But after the dinner, I managed to lose my phone. Stone cold sober. Long story, but someone who was at the dinner found it and brought it home for me. I retrieved it Monday, but managed to drop it in the toilet on Thursday. I've decided that perhaps this is HP's way of telling me I need to SLOW DOWN. Running like a lunatic trying to do too many things at once. I know I can't let my sobriety slip down my list of priorities though, and am trying to make sure I fit meetings into my chaotic schedule. I am lucky to have a sponsor who stays on my case about that.

Life is going to be chaotic and busy for quite some time with three kids under the age of 14, work, planning charity events, PTA events, writing a book, etc. In the melee, it's easy to lose sight of what's important. For me, that's my sobriety. Without that, there would be a very different kind of chaos. And it wouldn't be good at all. I can handle busy, but I've learned that I can't handle out-of-control, which is what happens when I drink. That's why the first step of Alcoholics Anonymous is perhaps the most important: "We admitted we were powerless over alcohol – that our lives had become unmanageable." Unmanageable just won't do.

Following the 12 Steps of AA helps us restore some order to our lives. The steps can bring back manageability. They can instill serenity. The eleventh step, "Sought through prayer and meditation to improve our conscious contact with God as we understood Him, praying only for knowledge of His will for us and the power to carry that out," helps immensely to bring us some peace. Through prayer and meditation, we can restore some semblance of order to our lives which had become utterly chaotic and unmanageable. The key for me is both remembering to pray and meditate and to make the time to do so. I always feel so much better when I do. Yoga helps immensely as well.

Chaos can make its way into everyone's lives at some point, whether one is an alcoholic or not. The key is how we deal with it and manage to restore order. I feel blessed to have the tools I have and the support of people around me to get back to a place where I can breathe and carry on. I'd write more but I've got a zillion things to do...

"Chaos was the law of nature;
order was the dream of man."

– Henry Adams, *The Education of Henry Adams*

CPSIA information can be obtained
at www.ICGtesting.com
Printed in the USA
FSHW020216010321
79017FS